AF365481

BURNOUT
TRUE SELF CALLING

Your chakra healing guide to burnout and finding your true self

By Claudia Andrea Reiter

CONTENTS

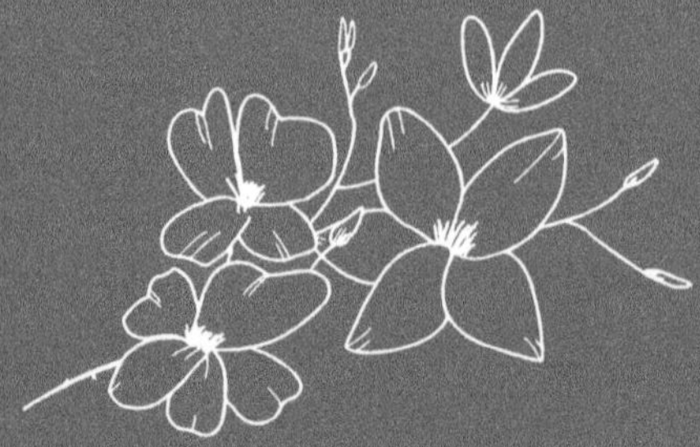

When I was a child, they told me I was not enough.

I was too small to reach for big things.

I was too little to understand.

I was too young.

I should not cry.

I should not be loud.

"I want to be a superhero one day", I said.

They laughed at me.

I was not old enough.

I was not good enough.

"Just wait until you are an adult", they said.

Now I am an adult.

I am too emotional.

I am an adult, and adults push through.

I have to be strong.

I should not cry. Adults don't cry.

I am a woman.

I must contain myself.

I should do what women should do.

I should get married and have children.

Why do I want a career?

I have to fit in.

What is wrong with me?

I am not pretty enough.

Nobody loves me.

I am too fat.

I don't know how I can ever be what they want me to be.

It is too much.

I need a break.

"Don't be weird", they said.

Nobody likes people who are different.

I have to fit in.

I want to be accepted.

I want to be loved.

I am not worthy of it.

I am not going to make it.

I am not good enough.

"Just wait until you are older", they said.

Then I grew older.

Don't do this, you are too old to do this.

Don't talk like this, you are no longer young.

Don't wear this, it is too young for you.

You can't do that. You are no longer good enough.

You can't learn something new. That is impossible.

...

This was where I started my journey.

I lived a life never being or doing what I truly wanted, because
at every stage in my life, I was told I was never enough. At the
same time, while I did everything they wanted, I lost myself.
I lost myself in the lie of never being good enough for others.
But I was good enough. There was always greatness within me.

So, I wasted a life. Believing a lie.

Stop wasting yours.

Awaken your true self.

Now.

MY BURNOUT STORY

From the outside, I looked like I had it all.

I was 29, married, living in a lovely flat, and working for a luxury brand climbing up the corporate ladder. On paper, I was achieving my personal goals. The truth, however, was very different.

My job as a product manager had become demanding and frustrating, and my marriage was falling apart. I was trying to keep the mask from slipping and do what I thought was expected of me: to be a good wife, a dutiful daughter, a loyal friend, and a high-performing employee. But that list, while admirable, completely ignored my own needs. The things Claudia needed to have the energy to push through the day and wake up in the morning refreshed, rather than drained and exhausted.

In the beginning, I tried to speak up and address my prob-
lems, but it was futile. And so, I kept doing what needed to be
done. I kept functioning. But something had to give, and it
was me.

Looking back, I can see now that the process of
burnout had been brewing for some time. I had
given away everything that was valuable to me:
time, energy, my heart and my health. I struggled
to find a moment of peace.

When under stress, I was easily agitated and emotionally
unstable. I was tense most of the time and the simplest thing
would send me over the edge. My phone running out of bat-
tery or my laptop playing up would send me into a spiral.

After frustrating meetings at work, I would flee to the bath-
room and cry. I felt like I couldn't cope anymore. I just wanted
it all to stop. But somehow, I was able to keep going, as if I was
on autopilot. When I got home at the end of the day, I would
pass out on the sofa straight away. I felt constantly fatigued. I
lacked the energy to exercise or meet with friends. Talking to
them or even just listening to them would drain my energy.
Weekends were the worst. Life felt meaningless, and I dread-
ed Sundays because I knew that the next day the hamster
wheel of my unfulfilling life would start all over again.

As I approached my thirties, I realised my marriage was over, and in 2020, I filed for divorce. Despite this hardship that comes with the end of a marriage, I continued to work in a job I no longer liked. I had been furloughed for a short while during the pandemic, but once I returned, the workload intensified. I was working even longer hours and my stress levels went through the roof. No matter how hard I tried, I couldn't unwind. I was under constant stress, day and night.

Soon, nights became my battleground. I couldn't fall asleep. My brain was working overtime, whirring and ruminating for hours on end. Thinking. Analysing. Constantly questioning. I just could not switch off. Every two hours I would wake with a start, gripped with panic. I was lucky if I managed to get four hours of sleep a night. The knock-on effect was that each day I felt worse than the day before.

All the things that I would usually rely on to help me, I had abandoned, believing I didn't have spare time for them. No yoga, no mediation, no walking in nature. I had reached what I now know was stage one of burnout: constant stress and inability to relax.

Soon I started to withdraw entirely from others – the second stage of burnout. I couldn't cope being around other peo-ple. I felt too weak, too exhausted to even speak. My tasks at work had no meaning anymore and I couldn't bear to engage with anything work-related. It all became pointless and insignificant. And so very soon I reached stage three of burnout – I started to de-personalise myself with everyone and everything around me. Depersonalisation is when a person feels removed from the unique qualities and features that make them feel special. It's the removal of an identity.

Between June and August, my life was little more than a blur. I felt like a robot fulfilling my duties alongside an endless stream of work, with no end in sight. What was even more worrying was the brain fog. I struggled to understand or take in what people were saying to me, either in work meetings or in personal conversations. I could hear words, but they didn't make any sense. I partly lost my reasoning capability, which was a frightening experience. But I didn't allow myself the time to investigate it further. "I have to keep functioning," was the mantra that pushed me forward.

I felt emotionally clouded and numb. I struggled to focus on work and began to make mistakes, which in turn made me more stressed. Friends told me that I sounded manic and chaotic when I spoke to them on the phone, as if I was being chased and on the run. I didn't understand what they were trying to tell me. I had tasks to do, expectations to fulfil.

I have one vivid memory of a Sunday afternoon when I was lying in bed, unable to move. My limbs were heavy, and I was crying silently; deep in my soul I just felt pain. I told myself "I don't want to work tomorrow." I realised how much I couldn't stand my job and all the meaningless demands of it. I felt so weak, so empty and dead inside. Any sort of task would be too much to cope with in that moment. I lived with my parents when I was going through my divorce, and even my lovely mum asking what I would like to eat overwhelmed me.

Then, on Monday 6th August at 7:10 am, I opened my work laptop after drinking my fourth coffee of the day. I read the first email of the day, tears began running down my cheeks. I began sobbing and crying uncontrollably. The breakdown had arrived.

I felt helpless and unable to cope any longer. The email was harmless; it was an inquiry about a product from a colleague, but I couldn't answer it. I felt like I didn't know anything any-more. My brain had gone blank. I was terrified and I couldn't understand what was happening to me.

Then, for the first time in my life, I paused.

I gave up on constantly pushing myself to the max. I had been doing it for too long. Ironically, I was working as a free-lance coach, supporting people with limiting beliefs and stresses. I had all the tools at my disposal, but even I had not been able to see my own crisis coming.

Eventually, I realised I needed help. So, I went to the doctor who diagnosed me with a severe stress disorder, which is more commonly known as burnout. They gave me a sick note for six weeks off work – but no further help, no further information. I tried to access a psychotherapist, but the waiting list was up to one year. After two weeks, I found a psychotherapist who was able to provide me three hours of therapy, but I gladly took them. She helped me understand what was going on in my life.

With her direction, I came to learn the following:

1. Burnout is a slow process and there are various stages to it.
2. Burnout needs time to heal and will not disappear after six weeks.
3. Burnout is not depression, although you might feel like it is.
4. Burnout does not only occur in the workplace, it can also happen at home.
5. Burnout can severely damage your brain. Chronic stress can reduce the size of your prefrontal cortex which is the area of your brain responsible for memory and learning.
6. Many people don't understand burnout.
7. The healing journey is hard work.
8. Our health service does not have the capacity to provide the support people with burnout need.

As much as my parents loved and supported me, they just couldn't understand how their daughter, who had always been such a powerhouse, could become so utterly powerless. At work, people tried to be sensitive, but after six weeks off, I was still not ready to cope with more than a few hours a day. But, due to the nature of the business, this was not always possible, and within three weeks of my return I had a recurrence of burnout. It was then that I decided I had to leave my job and take time off to heal and recharge my batteries for as long as needed.

I began researching and came to understand what burnout is and what I needed to do to recover holistically and sustainably. My journey to my inner self incorporated wisdom from ancient traditions like yoga, qigong and energy healing, as well as modern psychotherapy and introspection.

I could tell I was getting better when I began to enjoy being in nature again. I could laugh again. After yoga practice, I was also able to feel inner peace again. For the first time in months, I slept for a straight six hours and I knew this was a turning point on my road back to health. As the weeks went by, I felt more energised, and I was able to focus and concentrate enough to read books once again. Throughout my gradual recovery I learned more about burnout, and I realised how much more education everyone needs on the recognising its signs and how to provide sustainable stress management.

My recovery took me 10 months. Within this time, I practised a lot of energy healing, yoga, meditation and deepened my education on holistic healing practices. I trained in mediumship and developed my psychic abilities further in order to be able to help others, but also to know myself better. I followed my inner wisdom – my true self. Becoming who I am meant to be and truly am.

I became passionate about helping others and wanted to provide healing support and tools to help with extreme stress and burnout prevention. Help people finding their way home to themselves.

This led me to set up my own healing practice with my business partner, to assist people in healing and transforming holistically. Too many of us believe life is a treadmill and something to 'get through' – and I used to be one of those people. It was only when I reached rock bottom that I began to see how ill I was.

For me, 2020 was a year of crisis, but also of transformation. The thought of leaving my marriage, my job, and my home country in the space of just a year would have terrified me before, but I now see that it was what I needed to learn to live life on my terms. A life led by my true self.

PART 1: REFLECTION

There will be a day that you will, and you must follow your heart and self-expression. Burnout will occur and come back again until you step into your light.

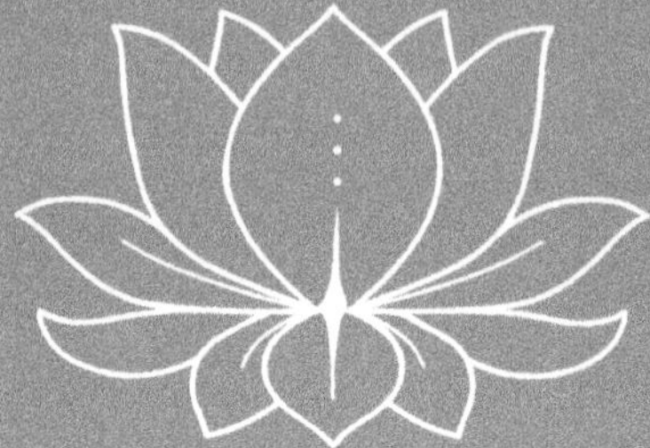

My yoga teacher once told me a lovely story. During teacher training, one of my classmates asked about how to deal with heavy struggles in life. The yogic scriptures teach us ways, but she was finding it hard to cope, especially when very bad things happen like losing a job, grieving the death of a loved one, a breakup or a health scare. How can someone see the good in life when things go terribly wrong?

"Life is like the journey of a lotus," our teacher said.

"Without mud, there is no lotus. Without the tough times in life, there is no life. It is all part of the journey. Sometimes we must go through the dark times, as must the lotus when it grows through the mud, in order to evolve, learn and become stronger and wiser."

This story is relatable. We are so often scared of the dark, of negative feelings, of the tough times – so much so that we forget that they are simply a part of life, a part that can help us unfold our true selves. Some needed a health crisis, in order to change their nutrition and lifestyle. Others needed to endure an abusive relationship, or poverty in order to find the strength to strive for betterment and come into their strength.

In every darkness lies a lesson for us to be learned. Can you see the lesson?

For me, burning out was a personal crisis that then led me to find and awaken my true self. Once we stop resisting the ups and downs of life, the impact of the darker times will lessen too.

But what does it mean to flow with life? What does it mean to live a life in congruence with your heart's wisdom?

In this book, I invite you to engage with my healing story from burnout, and the journey I took to find my way home to my true self by diving into my energy system, healing my chakras and restoring my lifeforce.

I believe that only once you are living your true self, will you find lasting health and happiness in all areas of your life. As an energy healer, I found that taking the journey through the chakra system not only brought them back into balance but took them to the next level. This is what unleashes your full potential; it not only heals the parts of yourself you have forgotten, but also lifts your true self to the surface.

As the lotus flower made her journey through the mud, I will take you on the journey from the bottom of your energy system up into your heart centre – your seat of your soul. Along the way you will find my personal stories, chakra insights and tools that will help you on your own spiritual journey through the chakra system and home to your true self.

Burnout is the signal to start our healing journey. The moment when your energy system collapses and is ready to be restored from the bottom up. A calling that our true self is ready to come out and take over, and for us to stop living a lie that drives us into the ground.

OUR ENERGY SYSTEM

Our energy system is so much more than just the seven chakras we learn from yogic teachings. It is worth mentioning that the chakra system has shifted over the time and new chakras, that are only a few hundred years old, have appeared to help us deal with the modern world.

I teach in my energy healing courses the whole system, however, explaining our energy body and its system alone could fill an entire book, therefore, I will focus only on the seven main chakras. On my healing journey I found that I could change my life, recover from burnout, restore my lifeforce and awaken my full potential by working on these alone.

"Chakra" is Sanskrit and means wheel, vortex or disk. They are lined up alongside our spine in the human body and each one is responsible for supplying energy to specific organs. While the meridians – think of them like energy vessels throughout the body – transport energy to the organs, the chakras infuse the meridians with energy. Any blockage within the meridians or chakras can lead to pain (i.e. headache), illness (i.e. depression) and imbalance (i.e. hormones), affecting our physical, mental, emotional and energetic health. Each chakra also governs specific emotions such as: transcendence, intuition, self- expression, love, identity, creativity and survival.

There are also energy layers around our bodies called the aura. Depending on which emotional and mental state we are in, we can radiate a particular energy.

Before diving into what burnout is, and how it occurs, first we must understand the basic anatomy of the chakras, focusing on our seven main bodily chakras. However, this is not a classic chakra book that guides you from the bottom to the top of the chakra system. Our chakra system is dynamic and interconnected, and it uses pairs as complementary energy centres, allowing for powerful energy metabolism. I believed for so many years that chakras stood alone, each working for themselves on parts of the body and individual areas, but this is not the case. During my psychic training I learned that they are complementary to each other and are all working collaboratively.

THE SEVEN CHAKRAS

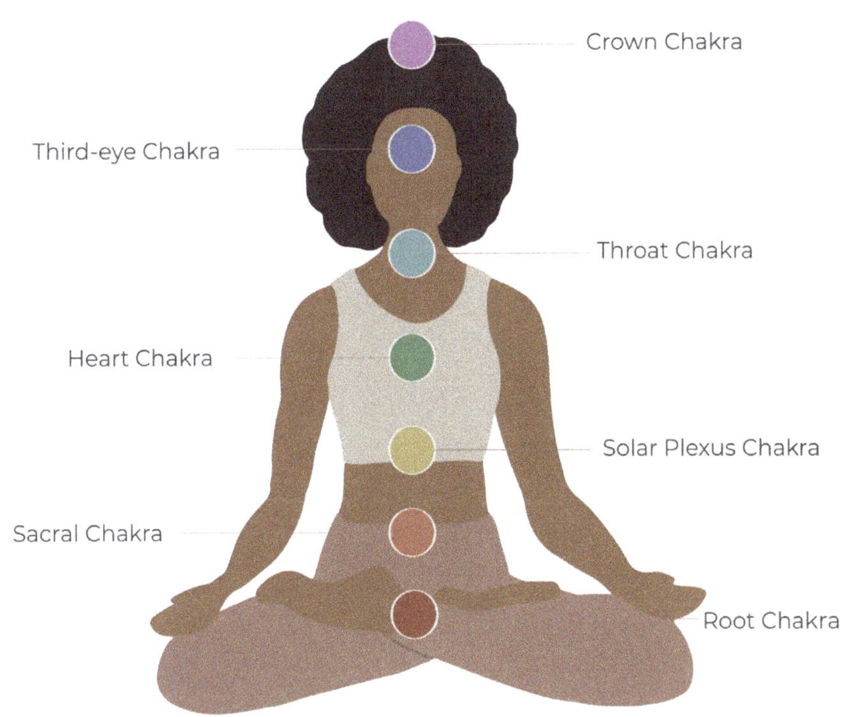

They are:

- THE ROOT AND CROWN CHAKRA: Addressing the needs of humanness and enabling us to create visions and live our spirituality. It enhances our connection to the universe, and to earth.
- THE SACRAL AND THIRD EYE CHAKRA: Creating the balance between thinking and feeling and reconnecting the body and mind.
- THE SOLAR PLEXUS AND THROAT CHAKRA: Finding your inner voice and living in your personal power.
- THE HEART CHAKRA: Living a soul-led life, healing and awaken your personal superpower.

You will find details of the interconnection of the complementary chakra pairs and lifestyle interventions and tools to restore balance, heal and let go while embarking your journey home to your true self.

Different sections of the book will cover the responsibilities of each chakra, as this is crucial for the understanding of how we can heal from burnout and understand how we got to the place where burnout could occur. As chakras are working tightly together, I will introduce you to the complementary chakra theory as well as highlighting the topics that are relevant to burnout healing and prevention. Each chapter has dedicated healing and lifestyle interventions for the chakras. In order to avoid writing an enormously long book, I have focused on topics of the chakras that are relevant to your healing journey of burnout or its prevention and how to awaken your true self and come into your light.

Just reading through the topics that each chakra covers, you might see some relationships between them, then you will better understand why they work in complementary ways rather than as a single energy unit.

IDENTIFYING BURNOUT

The World Health Organization defines burnout as a syndrome that occurs as a result of chronic workplace stress, especially when this stress is not well managed. It is characterised by three main points: the person feels like their energy is depleted and they are exhausted, they experience negative feelings or cynicism about their job, and they feel unable to carry out the functions of that job effectively.

But burnout can cause a deeper, more internal crisis, often forming as a result of not living the truest version of yourself, of not living as the person who you truly are but hiding behind a mask. Constantly suppressing your true nature costs your body and mind a lot of energy. It causes our batteries to empty, our holistic system to disconnect, and our mind-body-soul dynamic to become out of sync.

SYMPTOMS AND SIGNS

Recognising the signs of burnout can be difficult, particularly because burnout develops over weeks or even months, but it doesn't show up out of the blue. Symptoms can vary from person to person, but the following psychological symptoms are frequently present.

- Reduced performance and productivity
- Tendency to make mistakes
- Forgetfulness
- Anxiety
- Detachment from others and one's job
- Low mood
- Listlessness
- Difficulty concentrating
- Lack of creativity
- Lack of energy
- Fatigue
- Negative attitudes towards one's co-workers or job
- Low commitment to the role
- Loss of purpose
- Absenteeism
- Depressive mood
- Quickness to anger
- Cynicism
- Emotional numbness
- Frustration

Physical symptoms of burnout can show as:

- Exhaustion
- Muscle tension
- Headaches
- Gastrointestinal disorders
- Hypertension
- Difficulty sleeping or disruptive sleeping cycles
- Weakened immune system

KEEPING SCORE

The first step is to assess your lifestyle and risk of burnout by identifying your stress score. Chronic stress is the core reason for burnout, so it is important to know how much of a stress-led lifestyle you currently lead.

Rate the following areas of your life by how much they affect your well-being. You can rate them between 1 and 10, with 1 meaning it doesn't impact you at all, and 10 meaning it is a highly stressful area that has a significant impact on your life.

___ physical stress

___ mental stress

___ unhealthy eating patterns

___ unhealthy food (sweets, ready meals)

___ uncontrollable hunger

___ increased sensitivity of senses

___ deficit of vitamins and minerals

___ medication

___ brain fog

___ insomnia/sleeping issues

___ digestive issues

___ tiredness, lack of energy

___ moodiness

___ emotional instability

___ excessive caffeine consumption

___ lack of physical movement

___ negative self-talk

___ dehydration

___ shallow breathing

___ extreme weight gain or weight loss

___ issues of coordination and balance

___ increased pains and aches

___ lack of oxygen and clear fresh air

___ forgetfulness

Add up the numbers to find your total score: ______________

The lower the score the better, but a high score (over 120) indicates that you need to take action to reduce your stress levels. It is good practice to update your score every month or so and compare how you are developing and what you should focus on.

THE VIRUS OF THE WORLD

"Materialism leads us to lose awareness of our inner life, which is bad enough: but to be hypnotized by our own feelings and sensations and forget about others and the world around is worse."
From the Upanishads.

Burnout is a chance to pause and reassess your life, because something is clearly not going well. If you were to be honest with yourself, do you sometimes feel like you live to please others? Do you know what you want, or who you truly are? What brings you joy? What do you really like doing? Are you happy most of the time, or are you rarely happy at all?

We have become part of a society that endures long-term pain with the expectation that short-term pleasure will relieve us from it. We survive the long working week, all while waiting for the weekend to bring us the little pleasure of a break. This is where we give to short-term pleasure – if we even have the energy for it. For the most part, many of us just sleep, catch up on chores and admin, and waste hours on social media, then we end up exhausted every Sunday, dreading yet another week of work.

Cases of depression, burnout and even suicide are increasing worldwide. Thanks to the COVID-19 pandemic, even more people are stressed and on the verge of burnout. A study by Walters People (2021) reported that 47% of managers feared their employees were at risk of burnout upon returning to the office after working from home for so long. We all are at risk of just running into another mental health pandemic, and we may be already in the middle of it.

I often ask myself, where are we going as a society? Because I am scared when I look around and see the direction, we are heading in. Many of us have lost our sense of individuality; we define ourselves with material things and by comparing ourselves to others. Our social status, be it virtual or in-person, often matters more to us than our true feelings. Our number of social media followers means more than the number of true friendships we have.

We ignore the power of our intuition and numb our true selves to be socially accepted and liked. We jump into the hamster wheel, running constantly, wanting more, wanting things faster, and we lose ourselves in the process.

We have reached a stage where we are more comfortable lying to ourselves than we are with confronting how we feel. We answer the question "how are you today?" robotically with "I'm fine", although we might be suffering internally.

We desire change but are too terrified of what people would say if we declared what our dreams were, and if we tried to achieve them. So, we continue suffering quietly, gratefully accepting occasional pleasure and enduring long-term pain.

But we should be aiming for the opposite. We should be aiming for short-term pain, which is unavoidable in life, all while reaching for our dreams. It might be painful for us to face opposition from others, uncomfortable questions, and rejection, but taking a stand for what we genuinely want and who we truly are is worth it.

Any form of change takes us out of our comfort zone, but that is what is needed to evolve. The unfortunate truth is that the unhappiness and pain many of us feel in our lives is not strong enough to push us towards change. Instead, we wait for that moment. That moment of someone passing away. That moment where the doctor tells us that we have diabetes, cancer or any other disease. That car accident. The break-up. And even then, for some, that form of pain is still doesn't inspire them to make the change needed. For others, it sparks the fire to drastically change their current life around and live a life transformed for ultimate love, health and happiness. Burnout can also be that moment, but that moment can happen at any time, for any reason.

Burnout brings a health crisis to your door. It's an alarm that tells you to stop living your life this way and change, for the sake of your well-being, health, and your own happiness.

Imagine you are 90 years old. You are lying on your death bed. Now imagine that from today, you have not changed anything in your life. You have lived as you have done so far. All those dreams you've had have not been realised. How do you feel? What does this image do to you?

I don't want to depress you, that is not what this book is for. While this is a dark, morbid exercise, it serves a purpose. It wakes you up. You don't need life-threatening illnesses, an accident or other bad news to start changing your life for the better. To get out of your comfort zone. Lean into that feeling when you picture your 90-year-old self, and ask yourself this, do you want to keep living your life as you do now?

Burnout is a sign that it is time to breakout of the societal conditioning you grew up with. You need to stop living for others and take your superpower back, which was taken from you when you were a child and every day since then.

You were instructed on how to live, and you were told the expectations you had to live up to. This pressure is something that many people are not able to break free from, but it is possible. You must get in touch with what you want. Not what your parents, media, social media, friends or partners want. What you want.

Many people find it too uncomfortable to face their truth. They find it too hard to speak out what they would love to do, or to choose their own needs and wants over someone else's. But ignoring your own instincts initiates the numbing process. It instigates self-sabotaging behaviour. It can cause you to overeat, overconsume, overspend, overindulge in short-term pleasures like sex, parties, food, alcohol and drugs, and end up in a cycle that sends you spiralling downwards, further away from who you are.

Many people's lives are dictated by fear, and fear is dis-empowering judgmental and fills us with self-doubt. We understand that being an individual matters, but we must simultaneously be careful not to be too different. This is the catch.

As an individual, we have so much choice and everybody can be different, but most of us don't choose to show our full array of coloured feathers. We are too scared to be different. Too scared of being rejected. And if you are too different, all of a sudden you don't fit in. We need a system that empowers instead of destroying us.

Your free will is being buried, and burnout is one of several examples where your true self is being suppressed. You would not be in a personal crisis if you felt free to be who you truly are.

The illusion that success equals freedom is another trap. People believe they are free, but many of them are bound to an external presence – whether that's in person or online. And it's relentless, they barely can take a break. The responsibility to entertain and serve their followers is too big. Once again, they become bound by the expectations of others.

It's good to wonder about freedom, and free will, and if they even exist at all. There are rules and laws that have their reasons for keeping the world in order, but when you think about how you feel about yourself, are you free? Or are your actions, behaviours and thoughts based on a script written by someone else, so that you can be socially accepted by others. Are you eating when you are hungry, or eating when it is socially acceptable to eat? Are you putting on make-up and wearing clothes as a form of self-expression, or is it something you do in order to fit in and look good for others? Are you working out and going to the gym because you deserve health and a long life, or are you doing it to look a certain way for someone else? Do you do the things you do because you truly want to do them, or are you doing them to please others in order to receive love, acceptance, and confirmation?

It is a very unique and interesting currency we use to pay for our health. I believe we have a chance to gain personal freedom, but we need to grow into our own power and believe in ourselves more than anybody else does. We need to shine in all of our colours, all of our feathers, and express the unique greatness each of us truly are.

Burnout is a crisis we can learn from. Many people suffer from burnout but go back to work after learning some stress management tools, and they try to continue as they were. Clearly there are tools to manage the daily life stresses better, but for how long can they keep you functional? The relapse rates are obvious, and at the end of the day, it's just bad stress management, right? Let me tell you, there is no such thing as bad stress management.

We were built with a stress response that serves a particular purpose, that is to keep us alive. We are not made to suffer chronic stress.

Training resilience does nothing worthwhile. The amount of stress is not being reduced. No, you want to train your body to be able to keep coping with high amounts of stress, which anatomically you are not supposed to endure over a longer period either way. Chronic stress is poison. So let me ask you: Do you need stress management tools where literally nothing changes on the root cause of stress nor the amount of it, or do we need the personal power to actually set boundaries and live a life where chronic stress is non-existent?

We need to have this conversation. I wonder how many people are suffering in silence because they might not understand what's happening to them, or that there are ways to live without stress dominating their lives. For a while, people can withstand stress, but the system will break eventually.

We need to learn to listen to our bodies, and if we don't seek help from others, then at least seek help for ourselves and make sure to find our unique set of tools that provide healthy relief. We need this rather sooner than later.

When our internal voice, which was once a whisper, becomes a siren, and symptoms of burnout are finally showing themselves, it is time to act. We might not be able to change society all at once, but we can change ourselves and thus give ourselves a chance to live a magnificent life as who we truly are.

I know you are ready for this journey to holistic and spiritual healing, and you can see the gift that burnout can be. You are no longer wearing a mask or playing a game according to society's rules. You have just arrived at the beginning of your journey to healing – and you're on your way to finding your true self. It is time for your uniqueness to rise and for you to take control back, ultimately following your destiny. Don't ignore this opportunity. This is your chance.

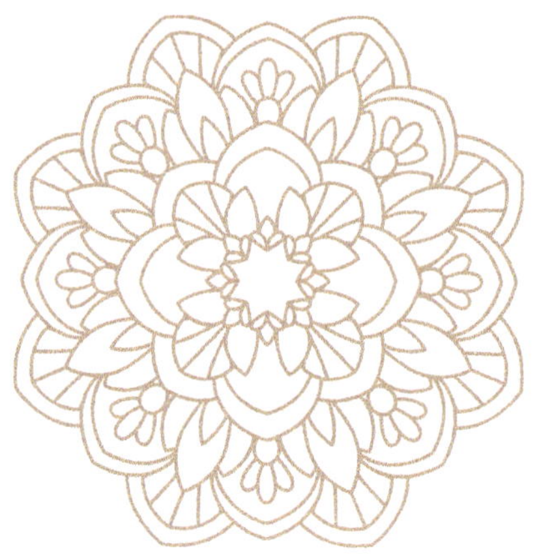

STRESS IS A PERSONAL CHOICE

We can decide if somebody or something stresses us or not. We are the only ones who have that personal power.

I know it's not necessarily what everybody wants to hear, but there is truth in this sentiment. You choose which lens you look through when you are given a situation. You can decide how it makes you feel depending on your inner scripts and mind-set.

When we look at burnout prevention, it is as much about healing and stress management techniques as it is about our minds, habits and beliefs that govern our thought system, our decisions-making and responses – both conscious and sub-conscious ones.

Let's take a classic workplace example. Maybe you woke up this morning feeling negative because last night you had a silly argument with your partner. You know it's silly, but you took that argument to heart and now you feel a bit off. You start your workday with a meeting and your boss seems on edge. When you ask a question, he snaps at you and answers it rather rudely. Your immediate reaction is to think "what did I do wrong?" This is when the stress response kicks in. Your mind spirals, endlessly thinking about what you could have done to trigger him. Did you make a mistake in the presentation you sent him last week? Did you forget to do something? Your brain takes off, desperately trying to find out what you did wrong, and this becomes your major concern. You're not even aware that your boss snaps at your colleagues in the same way.

You have two ways to respond to this scenario:

Option one: The lens of not being good enough.
You will look for faults on your end and experience fear that you messed up or did something wrong. As you keep believing you are at fault, your system experiences more and more stress.

Option two: The lens of understanding and compassion.
You don't pay further attention to your boss's response. You know you haven't done anything that warrants that kind of treatment. You wonder if your boss also had an uneasy evening the night before, or this morning. Some personal issues or pressure from the top management. Whatever it is, you know it has nothing to do with you and as such you don't take it personally.

REFLECTION MOMENT

Do you notice any particular patterns when you're thinking?

Are there moments when you are prone to overreacting and taking things personally?

What could you do to prevent that?

How do you treat yourself in such moments?

During a training session in yoga therapy for mental health I came across a very simple concept: stress is fear. Fear rules us. Fear keeps a society in check. Fear keeps us in check. Fear of not being good enough. Fear of being rejected. Fear of being alone. Fear of being different. Fear. Fear. Fear. Chronic stress is constant fear. Our bodily reactions are the same with fear as with stress. We are conditioned from childhood in a way that our instinctive stress response is no longer concerned about the safety of our livelihood but rather about others opinions, societal acceptance, and fitting in. In short: suppressing our true nature.

The core problem here is two-fold. We do not know how to change. We do not know how to love and trust ourselves. Listen inward to the wisdom within us. This leads to a distorted vision of ourselves, creating a negative impact on our mind, belief-system, and self-worth. But there is more to us than just our bodies and minds. We are also energy.

We have an energy system that keeps us functioning; it protects us so we stay fit and healthy and it helps us manifest our dreams into reality. However, if our energy system is distorted through stress, past trauma or unhealthy lifestyle choices, it can become imbalanced, and flow becomes blocked. This can manifest as physical illnesses, negative thinking patterns, self-destructive behaviour, burnout and many other symptoms. Therefore, we must take the healing journey through our chakra (energy) system.

My personal belief is that the best you can do for your physical, mental, emotional, and energetic health, is to be who you truly are. Most of us know that lifestyle plays a huge role in our overall health and wellbeing, yet it is sometimes difficult to maintain it. I've struggled in the past with weight, with emotional co-dependency, and with chronic stress.

The one thing that changed everything was becoming my true self. But what is the true self?

The true self is the awakened version of you, connected to your heart and essence. Being your true self is loving yourself unconditionally and taking care of yourself and your needs whenever needed. It's knowing yourself and knowing what sparks your light. You live your life in accordance with your values.

For many of us, the closest we've been to our true selves is when we were children. Remember when you weren't frightened that you might fall while climbing a tree? When you cried because you were hungry, or threw a tantrum because you were upset? Did you care about what people thought of you? Not really.

You were a fully feeling, being, experiencing the flow of your emotions, instead of being trapped inside a thinking machine. But then adults stepped in, and they told us what to do and how to feel. Teachers, friends, society got us caught up in a wheel of fulfilling expectations, of trying to please everyone but ourselves, of constantly being there for others, giving our time and energy away in order to pursue materialistic things, and becoming obsessed with status. We began living the life that was expected of us - believing it would bring us happiness.

HEALING BURNOUT HOLISTICALLY

Burnout can occur in other areas of our lives, not just in the workplace, so when overcoming burnout, several different areas require attention. You will find recommendations and exercises in each chapter of this book that will address all four areas below to support healing.

• Spiritually: Burnout is the suppression of your true self. Your soul yearns to finally break free from your cage and follow your bliss. You don't live according to your personal values, but according to the values of others.

• Energetically: Your energy is depleted and unable to restore itself over and over again. You need time off to rebuild your energy stores and create balance by doing things that support your energy system overall. Your chakra system needs a reload and your prana energy needs to be restored. Letting go of trauma or limiting beliefs can help release blockages in the energy system that supports healing on emotional, physical, mental and energetic levels.

• **Physically:** Your nutrient and vitamin depot is running low and your body takes every last bit of energy it can find to cope with the stress, causing fatigue. Chronic stress leads to adrenal fatigue, which again impacts your hormone system, sleeping, and overall physical performance. Your heart rate is constantly elevated, and your nervous system is under constant stress which can cause damage in brain cells and cardiovascular illnesses, among other health issues.

• **Emotionally and mentally:** Burnout causes you to become emotionally numb. You lack the energy to experience or express feelings and emotions. Your mind becomes clouded and unable to think; it is almost as if you freeze. Think of your mind like a car that has run out of petrol, but you keep on driving nonetheless. Now the engine is broken, and no amount of petrol will fix it. Instead, the engine itself needs attention. Finally, your emotional threshold to deal with stress has reached a shocking new low, which then leads to emotional instability. This is the reason for getting angry or crying over the smallest things.

REFLECTION MOMENT

Ask yourself these questions:

· You reached a particular age. Do you really want to be married, buy a house and have kids now?

· You have a well-paid job in a big corporation. Everybody admires you because you seem to be doing so well. Nobody knows that this job is the cause of your depression and is making you sick. Why do you stay? What is keeping you from changing? Does it matter what others think of you? Or don't you remember, or recognise, what your heart truly desires?

· You believe that you are too young or too old to do something that would excite you. Is this really your own, organic belief? Or has it been thrust upon you?

· You know you are not happy. Are you living to please others, or to please yourself?

· You have been told you are not good enough. Do you think this because you are reminded of it every day? Or, if left alone, do you realise it's not true? Do you believe you are good enough?

· What fears are running your life? Fear of being alone? Fear of not being good enough to go for your true desires. Become aware of your fear and inner scripts and reflect on how well did they serve you thus far?

· You are satisfied in your relationships. Are you truly happy or are you afraid of being alone? Are certain relationships preventing you from being your true self? Toxic relationships exist and can prevent us from coming into the truest version of ourselves. Ask yourself, are you attached to certain relationships that you know deep down are no longer serving you?

- Spend more time with yourself.
- Meditate.
- Go for walks in nature.
- Practice yoga, qigong, and tai chi.
- Read a book. A good place to start would be *A new Earth* by Eckart Tolle, *You Are A Badass* by Jen Sincero or *Light is the New Black* by Rebecca Campbell.
- Question yourself. Question your mind-set, thought patterns and responses.
- Pause actively and turn inward.
- Do the things that spark your inner light. If you don't know what that is, then take the time to remember. What were the things you loved doing when you were younger? If nothing much comes to mind, why not try something new? Do something you'd never have thought of doing and surprise yourself.

PART 2: BETWEEN HEAVEN AND EARTH

"Not everybody will understand your journey.
That's okay. You are here to live your life,
not to persuade others of your journey."
Bahar Yilmaz

WHEN YOUR TRUE SELF CALLS

For most of my life, I've operated like a machine. There were
things that needed to be done, expectations that needed to
be met, and I relentlessly pushed myself to be better, to do
more and to prove that I am good enough.

When I was 27, I would get up at 4am to prepare breakfast
and get ready for my two hours commute to work. I would
work all day and finish at 4pm. My way home was always a
painful journey because of traffic. Finally, once I was home, I
would cook, do the house chores, and eat. I'd be surprised and
frustrated that the day had passed without me having done
anything for myself.

I didn't tell my parents how hard it was to make ends meet. My
salary was a joke. Health-wise, I had reached my limit. I was sleep
deprived. My diet was a nightmare. My weight was unhealthy.
My mental health was devastated. This was when my first burnout hit home.

I did my best at the time. I chose to ignore it. However, I always had my trusty inner critic at hand that would keep pushing me. It kept me on autopilot and fed me thoughts that told me things would get better. Sometimes these thoughts were negative and destructive, but they ignited a fear inside me that kept me going and kept me suppressing my emotions. Keeping busy stopped me from thinking, from questioning myself, not giving my true self the chance to be taken seriously.

Soon I was broke. I wanted to quit my job, but I still had bills to pay. I was plagued with anxiety over money. Fear of not having enough money. How was I going to pay back my student loan? How was I going to have enough money to buy food?

My marriage sucked. "My husband thinks I am a loser," I told myself. He did not understand what it meant when the doctor said I was approaching early stages of depression. "You are weak," he said. "You have to get a thicker skin. You are too emotional." It hurt and the fear of not being good enough kept me pushing and trying to be strong.

Then I gained weight. All the stress from work and my marriage made me binge eat. It was comforting. I felt better, but only temporarily. "You should lose weight," my husband told me. "You are fat. You are not attractive like this." Leading to self-harming thoughts of "Who can love me looking like that? No wonder I am all alone. I do not deserve love."

I was alone. I was alone in a foreign country, and all my friends and family were far away. I had no one I could talk to. I was scared to talk to them at the same time, worries and fear about what they might think of me kept me suffering in silence.

I chose to continue fighting, but I was fighting against myself. I was not allowing my true self to speak. Never pausing or taking a break. Instead, I continued on autopilot. I chose to continue pushing and maintaining some sort of control over my life that was on the brink of falling apart, when all I wanted was to rest. I had to keep myself going, in order to keep everything going around me. I needed money, I needed my job, I needed acceptance from others since I couldn't accept myself.

I was holding onto the belief that if I kept pushing, I would keep this control, I would not lose myself, although I was already lost. But ignoring my human needs was not serving me. My true self was calling for help. Calling for me to stop. Calling for me.

What are you trying to control in your life? What are you holding on to for fear of otherwise falling apart? What does control give you, that you cannot give yourself?

TOPICS COVERED BY THE ROOT AND CROWN CHAKRAS

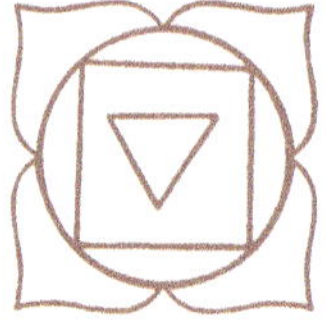

- Love of life on earth and fellow human beings.
- Self-love and self-respect and recognising your own needs.
- Inner safety and sense of security.
- Meeting basic needs and respect for your instincts.
- Stability.
- Acceptance and acknowledgment of your own time and speed with things, allowing yourself to rest.
- Connection to your animal instincts and brain.
- Ability to recharge and let go, as well as grounding to the earth.

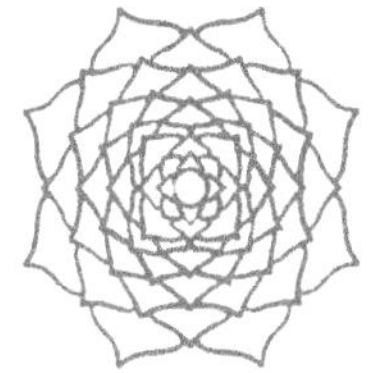

- Higher-self connection and higher-self healing.
- Connection to universal energy.
- Compassion and love for everything.
- Dedication and trust in life.
- Connection to spirit world.
- Spirituality.
- Accepting learning processes in life.
- Ability to live and experience the joys of life.
- Stepping out of the comfort zone.
- Having the courage to shine your light and show your uniqueness.

One of the biggest lessons I learned when working on my root and crown chakras was to respect and trust myself. Growing up, I was told how to be and what to do, and this not only kills the essence of who we truly are, but it also destroys our ability to respect and trust ourselves.

We never believe we are good enough, even if we know we had a great performance at school, or on the job, there is always a voice asking us why we didn't do better. I remember in school when I would get a B in an exam, I would be happy because my parents were happy to see me getting As and Bs.

One day, I came home and showed them my B in a maths exam, and my dad asked me why I could not make it an A.

I remember how sad and disappointed I felt, and I was questioning myself. Strengthening the belief of not being good enough.

This example in childhood carries over into adult life. We apply for a job and feel like we really nailed it, but when we don't get it, we feel like a loser, like we're not good enough. We are confident that our relationship is strong, and later we find out our partner let us down, betrayed us, and then it spirals down to losing more and more respect for ourselves.

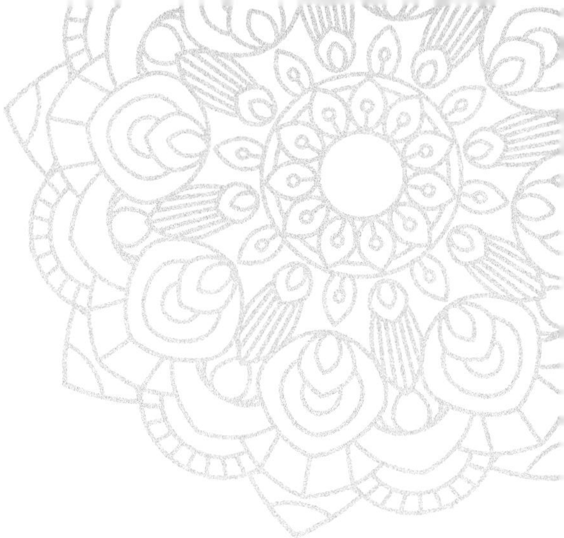

We end up doing anything and everything just to be loved and accepted by others. We do not believe that we even have the potential for greatness within us nor in our reach. We don't trust ourselves and seek constant validation from others. And in doing so, we actually accomplish these three things:

1. We bury the connection to our higher self and to our essence.
2. We shy away from shining our own light and give up on the belief that life is getting any better for us.
3. We completely ignore our human needs.

In order to start respecting our lives and ourselves again, we must set boundaries, stop the autopilot, let go of pleasing others, and listen inwards.

What does my body need right now? More sleep? A break? Movement? Answer these questions and give your body what it needs. What does your heart desire right now? Reading? Spending time with your loved ones? Traveling? Following and respecting your instincts and human needs, is important to create balance in your system.

If you constantly neglect your human needs, your skills and abilities, what you have will deteriorate. It's like the saying "what you don't use, you lose". Humankind has developed from a highly active species to inert and immobile beings. We don't use our bodies as much as we should to ensure lasting health. We barely think for ourselves, nor question the norms. We don't think critically, which prevents growth and evolution. We are letting machines and technology take over our thinking and do most of the work for us. We give the responsibility for our life away and when things don't work out in our favour, we blame others. The job, the government, our pet, the star constellation. It is easy, isn't it? But just because it's easy it doesn't mean it's right. We do a lot, just not taking ownership of our own life. However, that is what we need to do if we want to live a life worth living.

With the root chakra, you must also consider trust and time. Many of us have reached a high level of impatience, so if we don't get something immediately or see success instantly, we give up, or become stressed. Developing technology so it is constantly getting faster and more accessible has a detrimental impact on how we perceive time. Our primal instincts are unable to keep up with this new way of living and it brings our root chakra into distress.

Thank you, Amazon Prime, because if I can get that item by today, I rather pay a higher price than wait for shipment that will take a week.

If I don't lose six pounds after one week of this new diet, then this diet must be stupid and ineffective.

If customer service can't resolve the issue now, it is a rubbish customer service.

Our expectations are on an unrealistic level. If your business is not generating sales within the first three months, then your business has failed. We could all use a reminder that creation and success need time, dedication, and consistency.

The way we have developed as a society has turned us into successful, but self-sabotaging beings. We no longer give things or people time to grow and evolve, ad qualities like patience and trust have become rarities. Everything is now or never. We don't have faith in the process nor life. We want to be in control.

If we did trust in time, patience, and the process, we would feel okay about making lifestyle changes and seeing great results in four months instead of one week. We would enjoy working on our own business and giving it time to grow and become known. We might even improve in certain areas because we gave ourselves time to rethink, assess and improve. But instead, we beat ourselves up if things aren't successful immediately. Life should be about allowing yourself the time to create and evolve. About becoming comfortable sitting still and reading a book while things are developing on a discreet level.

If you give your all to something, wait and give it time. Later, return to it. See how you can improve or reap what you sowed.

This also gives you a chance to recharge. You need to stop and give yourself permission to rest.

Things need time to unfold their magic, you don't pressure a butterfly out of its cocoon. The butterfly comes out when it is the right time to evolve.

TRANSFORMING FEARS

If there is one emotion that runs our society it is fear. However, fear is not necessarily a bad emotion. Fear has a purpose: to keep us safe. Fear stops us from doing stupid things, like crossing a busy street full of traffic, jumping in front of a train, or going too close to the edge of a cliff.

But fear can also serve as a catalyst.

Sometimes fear motivates us to get something done. For example, before giving a big presentation you might be worried. You fear something going wrong, but this fear drives you to prepare and do the best you can to deliver a great performance. The fear of getting ill might motivate you to exercise, eat healthier and reconsider your lifestyle. Fear motivated me to make changes in my life and start living my life on my terms. The fear of not being allowed or able to follow my heart motivated me to quit my safe nine-to-five and start my own business while following my heart.

We are so scared of fear that we try to avoid looking at it and feeling it. According to my spiritual coach, if we want to let go of fear, we need to first own it. And this means feel into the fear. Feel it deeply, acknowledge its existence and then we can let it go. If we do not allow ourselves to feel into it and let it go afterwards, we can develop an addiction for fear and negative feelings. Which is dangerous as seeking constantly fear keeps us in place, in our comfort zone but it also gives us a false sense of the awareness of life.

Fear can both confine and empower us, it depends on how you look at it. If we are honest, fear is nothing but an emotion and emotions are energy. So, it depends on what you are using this energy for. You can stay put and don't actively create the life you want to live, or you use it as an energy booster to push through and go after your dreams. The choice is yours, but it can be a useful exercise to examine the kind of fear that dominates your life.

REFLECTION MOMENT

What is your biggest fear? What are you most afraid of?

Where does this fear originate from? What has happened to you in the past?

What does this fear try to protect you from?

How does this fear prevent you from living the life you truly want to live?

Do you want to let this fear prevent you from your dream life?

What can you tell your fear and yourself, so you no longer need protection from that fear?

THE POWER OF BEING 'HUMAN'

In the spiritual scene and in positive psychology, there is a lot of emphasis on love and compassion, and being positive. But at the same time, in everyday life we are expected to be in control of our emotions, to be rational, to be good but not too much of anything. Don't be childish, don't be loud, don't be different.

We have a full spectrum of emotions, and we don't get to pick and choose the ones we want to experience. We are human beings. Being human means that we will be loving at times, but also angry at times. We will get hurt and become sad, but only as much as we will be happy and joyful. We will be loud, and we will be quiet. We are allowed to be childish, and we can also be serious when the situation requires. We are not robots, despite the pressure to suppress our emotions. Following your heart, living a life, and being human incorporates the full array of emotions we are able to feel. So, embrace the being human part and don't shy away or feel bad if you feel something "negative".

When you are angry, then express it, release it, and come back to normal. When you are sad, cry for a while before you move on again. Own your emotions and then let them go. If you are reaching towards an ideal of being all sunshine and love twenty-four-seven, you are setting yourself up for failure. Look at little children as an example. There is no other being that changes and expresses its feelings and emotions as they do. Can you imagine little Jimmy getting told off by his mother and holding a grudge for the next ten years because he was not allowed to play with the neighbour child that one night? Of course not. Kids are master of living in emotional flow. Feeling everything and letting it go.

Be a human, take the good with the bad, and make sure to explore yourself. We are on earth for a damn short time, so make it worthwhile. Follow your human needs in order to rise spiritually, and then you can be spiritually strong. Being the most spiritual and truest version of yourself is the best for your mental, physical, emotional, and energetic health.

REFLECTION MOMENT

Are there rules, structures, or societal beliefs that you feel reducing the number of possibilities open to you?

Do they keep you from not reaching your full potential? How do they prevent you from living the life you genuinely want to live?

What rules or beliefs are they? How can you lessen their impact?

What can you choose to belief or do instead?

YOUR INNER DRIVER

Everybody of us has inner drivers. Inner drivers can also be called internal stressor enhancers. For example, they could be money, noise, your boss, people, or a particular smell that puts us in a state of stress. But then there are inner drivers that are more like thinking patterns or beliefs that 'drive us' and push us to act a certain way. The good thing is they help us get things done. The bad thing is that if they take over, they can lead to burnout. The following are a few examples of inner drivers:

Reoccurring negative thinking patterns and dramatising. You know you fall into this category if you use words such as 'never' and 'always' in the context of generalising negatively.

> Examples:
> - "I never experience true love."
> - "Nobody cares about me."
> - "No matter what I do, it is never enough."

Deficit thinking. If you always act and behave from a place of not having or being enough.

'Have to' thinking. When we believe we have to do or be something. For example, we have to go to work, we have to dress a particular way, we have to earn money, we have to get married before 30 etc.

Perfectionism. The desire to succeed on all levels.

Desire to be liked by others. Also known as the disease to please.

'I have to be strong' thinking. When we don't allow ourselves to show or feel weakness. In these cases, a strong desire for independence is sought.

Desire for control. This is a desire that is based on learned helplessness from childhood. People with this driver usually learned early on not to trust themselves.

Over emphasis on your inner driver will drive you into the ground, and even cause burnout, when not identified and transformed, and it always results in a disconnection between body and mind. Arguably, it even caused our society to be overly based on rationality, materialism and logic, and results in many people ignoring their hearts and body-mind connection. In order to work successfully with our inner driver and transform the energy connected with it, we must follow these three steps:

1. Identify your inner driver.
2. Understand where it originates from.
3. Learn new ways to use the energy of your inner drivers to your advantage.

One way of identifying your driver is by thinking of a situation that stresses you out. Then ask your-self, what is stressing you about this situation or person, and why? What is your inner monologue like? What words are coming up? Something like "I have to do this…", "If I don't do this, people will think less of me…"? The words you use to talk to yourself can give you a great hint of what your inner driver is.

Inner drivers are limiting beliefs that rule our life on various levels. There is a very powerful exercise to identify such limiting beliefs and turn that limiting belief into your most beneficial thought. The following questions will help you to identify them, but they will also provide a counter measure to help turn them around, and transforms them into something empowering for you, so that they help you rather than drive you into the ground.

Step 1: What was the earliest most painful event you remember in your life?

Step 2: How did this event make you feel? Can you describe the feelings and emotions you had back then?

Step 3: What about that situation hurt you the most?

Step 4: What did this painful experience make you believe about yourself, about your life or about others?

Step 5: Reality check: is this belief really true? Can you be 100% certain that this is true? What proof do you have?

Step 6: How do you feel with this belief now?

Step 7: Can you turn this belief around? For example: "I am always alone" can turn into "I am never alone".

Step 8: How does this new alternative sound to you? How does it make you feel? Can you find proof that this alternative is true?

In the end, ask yourself if you can accept this new alternative as your new truth. Can you see that the old limiting belief doesn't serve you any longer and actually never has? Can you see a learning opportunity or a lesson in what that experience made you become? Did it make you stronger, or more independent?

THE MYTH OF 'COMFORT AND SAFETY FIRST'

One of the reasons why we sometimes resist change is that our reptilian brain – the very old part of our brain which is responsible for our instincts and basic needs being met – is driven by the rule: 'comfort and safety first'.

'Comfort and safety first' means we need to stay safe, and we should always find the easiest way out with least resistance. But if you decide to make some bigger life changes, like finally doing the things you want, making yourself a priority, quitting your current job and start something completely different or travel the world, that rule comes into conflict. And if you want to exist in harmony, you don't want any resistance getting in the way of it. But this is a learned behaviour that needs to be overcome.

We have developed this system based on our past experiences. Touching a hot stove once tells us that we shouldn't do it again. So, the same goes for experiences with a particular job, with a particular change you once made and maybe something went wrong, or any instance when you have been hurt, emotionally or physically. Therefore, a negative experience is saved in our memory or subconsciousness.

If you haven't changed much in your life, perhaps it is because you grew up according to the norm. Perhaps you followed set rules, so you rarely initiated change. Perhaps you learned from others that change is dangerous or that it could have negative consequences.

The 'new' also means the unknown, and so we allow fear to sit in the driving seat of our decision-making process, and change is not pursued because we'd rather stay safe with what we know and can control than risk something else. We'd rather stay in a comfortable place than have to struggle with personal growth, learn new things and face potential failure.

Therefore, we self-sabotage our potential and ourselves by staying in the comfort zone, and we avoid change at any cost. This system was created by three things: by our past experiences, by the environment we grew up in, and our belief system about the world and about ourselves. How can we reverse this process? By changing the way we think about ourselves, and start seeking out our true identities.

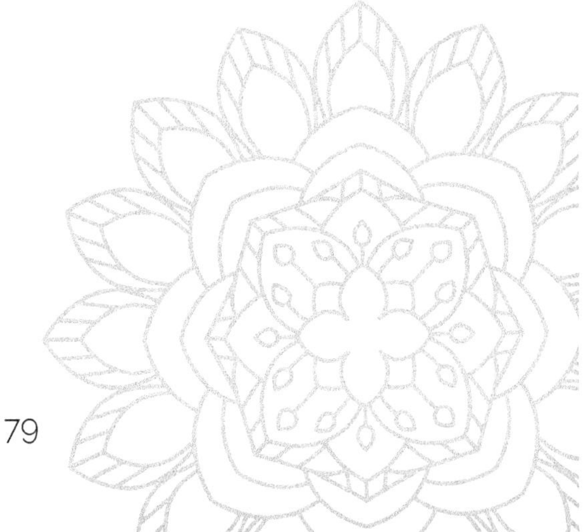

LASTING CHANGE

For any lasting change to happen, we have to become aware of what is currently not serving us and gain clarity on what we truly want. The great neuroscientist Dr. Joe Dispenza wrote an amazing book called *Breaking the Habit of Being Yourself*. What was so exciting is the science behind it. It explains how thoughts create your life and how you perceive it. Try to examine the thoughts you think, and you might find that ninety percent of your thoughts are the same as the day before.

What does that mean? It means that, day-to-day, we are not changing. We are reliving each day again and again. The same thoughts lead to the same choices. The same choices lead to the same experiences. The same experiences lead to the same emotions. The same emotions drive our neurochemistry and genetic expression. This means that our thoughts create our life. If we want to change, we must start with our thoughts first in order to change our choices, emotions and experiences.

We cannot change if we stay the same person. This means we must change our thoughts and emotions to produce new behaviours and experiences. When these new beliefs are established, behaviours become the new habits of the new version of who you want to be; the beliefs become ingrained in your brain and body. This is how real change can take place.

We are what we think. But also, we can change who we are by changing what we think and what we feel about ourselves. This is the blueprint to lasting change.

The science behind it is called neuroplasticity: the brain's own ability to reorganise its neuronal structure and build or rebuild new, strong neuronal connections. This is hugely beneficial when adapting to new situations or new environments. Neuronal connections that are not being used or reinforced through repeated experiences or emotions get smaller and smaller until they no longer exist – this is also called neuronal pruning. Other neuronal connections are reinforced with constant repetition of doing the same things or feeling the same emotions, and they grow bigger and stronger.

How can we use this to our advantage? If we alter our thoughts, and in doing so alter our emotions and begin behaving differently, we are practicing change and forming a new identity. Though we might practice these new feelings and experiences in our heads first, before we experience them in reality, we are already altering our brain structure and creating new neurological connections. By creating those new ones, we weaken those that no longer serve us, and in doing so we create a new person, and lasting change can occur.

After a while, you will be able to identify your limiting beliefs and inner drivers and turn them around, transforming them into the thoughts about yourself that are the most beneficial. You can start integrating this new thought into your daily life by saying it aloud or in your head. Visualise yourself doing and feeling this new thought and incorporate it into your daily routine. Practice this over and over again, and eventually you will become a new version of yourself.

YOUR NEW IDENTITY

An important model I would like to introduce is the identity loop, designed by German bestselling author, coach and pod-caster, Laura Malina Seiler. This loop is also quite a nice visual to what Dr. Joe Dispenza described in his books. Our identity is our belief system, determined by our thoughts, feelings, and actions. Therefore, it is important that we become aware if our current identity is serving or sabotaging us.

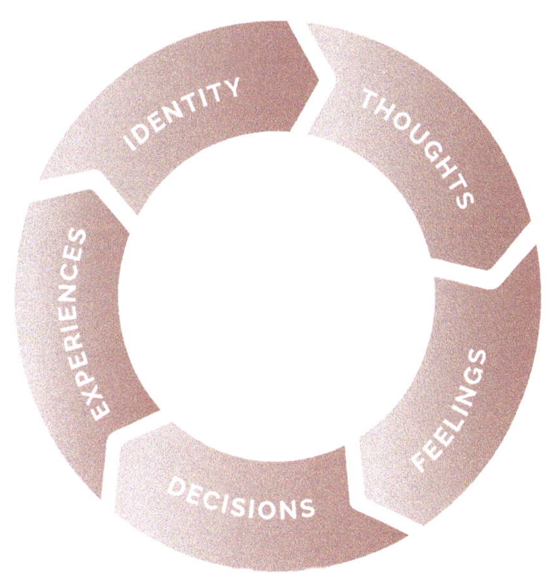

For example, if you identify with the belief "I am ugly", then your thoughts become based on that core belief, and manifest as something like "I will never find a partner," "I will stay single forever," I can't wear nice things," and "nobody likes or will ever love me because I am ugly." This results in deeper feelings of loneliness, shyness, being afraid, a lack of self-worth, body hate and a lack of confidence. Such feelings then impact our decision making. We are too terrified to take bold decisions. We would rather choose not to ask someone out, not wear something colourful, not apply for a particular job or not speak up in a meeting.

Based on these decisions, we begin to experience negative things that just confirm our limited beliefs and identity. We are lonely, single, we don't wear nice clothing, we struggle with body weight, we don't go out and meet friends, we don't work in that fancy job. Can you see how a core thought like "I am ugly" can go on to rule your mind, thoughts, feelings, decisions and experiences? Other examples of core beliefs are: "I am not intelligent," "I am dumb," "I am not good enough," "nobody loves me," "I am not worthy of love," and "I am lonely."

Following the identity loop, can you go inward and create a status quo of your current identity loop? What is your core belief about yourself? i.e. I am dumb, not lovable, not good enough, intelligent, awesome, full of potential?

Tune in and see what is your core belief and then analyse for yourself, what thoughts are you thinking based on this core belief you have?

Go one step further and reflect on what feelings are you feeling based on those thoughts? Can you see what kind of decisions you took because of the thoughts you were thinking and the feelings you were feeling? Do you realize the experiences you went through because of the identity you created for yourself?

Once we realize the power our beliefs hold over us, we can take the next step and create slowly a new identity.

The great thing is that we can change our identity and core beliefs using the exercise we just did before. Identify your core belief and inner driver about yourself and turn it around. You already identified your inner driver and turned it around to your most beneficial thought. Let's go one step further and do the same thing with your core belief, your identity.

You just went through the identity loop above with the limiting core belief about yourself. Now, let's have a look who you want to become.

STEP 1 - your identity

Who do you want to be? i.e. good enough, worthy of love, intelligent, an entrepreneur, an author, a loving mother…
Make sure you start with the powerful words of I AM.
For example: I am healthy and fit. I am beautiful.

STEP 2 - your thoughts

What thoughts would you be thinking based on your new identity?
Example: I love to move my body and eat healthy. I am fit and love to take care of me. Everyday a bit better than yesterday. I can do this. I deserve health and happiness. I love my body.

STEP 3 - your feelings

What feelings would you be feeling?
Example: Energised, upbeat, confident, sexy, strong

STEP 4 - decisions

What would you have to do daily to feel and think as the person you want to become?
Example: Wear clothes I love and feel good in them, exercise regularly, sign up to a gym or fitness class, choose healthy food options, sleep enough, do the things that make me happy

STEP 5 - experience

What experiences would you be making based on your new identity?
Example: Meet people who share the same passion as me, wonderful fit friends, a healthy and fit body, love, feel good in my clothes, attract more health and joy, go on a date, do a job I love.

Becoming aware that we always have a choice is very powerful. An inner driver or core belief will not be replaced or disappear overnight, but you have taken the first step, and from now on you can choose your new loving action and over time you can transform and turn your life around completely.

SELF-SABOTAGE

When we are trying to change our habits, and wanting to better ourselves, we sometimes hit some roadblocks or our subconscious tries to prevent us to change. When we are stuck in this self-destructive stress cycle, where our inner drivers or limiting beliefs are in the lead, where we constantly lie to ourselves and struggle to do the things that are good for us, then we are doing one thing that will keep us in this cage: self-sabotage.

We believe what we do is based on our free will, when really we are acting based on our inner driver and we are being led by fear of what will happen if we don't do what our inner driver pushes us to do. So, you can see there are two things that create the circumstances that can lead to crisis.

1. Our inner driver (based on childhood beliefs or trauma) and thus resulting in,
2. Fear

Let's have a look at your own self-sabotaging behaviour only if you become aware of what you are doing, you can initiate lasting change.

· When do you feel like you are forced to do something? Not freely, but rather doing something because you feel you have to, although you don't want to do it?

· How do you feel in such moments physically, mentally, energetically, and emotionally?

· What self-sabotaging tools are you using in order to not change and prevent yourself to coming into your personal power?

· Food is something many of us use to cope with the things we don't want to face. Do you use food to distract yourself or numb particular feelings? Do you punish your body with food, either by overeating or not eating at all?

· Do you use other substances to numb your feelings?

· Where in your life do you build, intentionally or unintentionally, walls around yourself? Are you scared of change, the new or the unknown? Are you even scared of your own power?

· What is the major benefit for you to not change?

THE STRUGGLE OF SELF-LOVE

You are deserving. You are deserving of a fulfilled and happy life, full of good health and love. We are on this earth to live a life filled with adventure, experiences, happiness, and love. However, the society we grow up in is the only reason why we tend not to believe that we are deserving of good things. The same goes with the classic belief that most of us have: the belief of never being good enough.

But can you accept and integrate into your system that you will never be good enough – and that is absolutely, okay?

Another reason for our suffering is the constant chase of proving to others and ourselves that we are good enough, as well as seeking the stamp of approval from others that validates us. We have lost our sense of self-worth and self-love.

But the question of being good enough is an illusion. The truth is you are born good enough, otherwise you wouldn't be here. A footballer does not become a pro overnight. He was born with basic skills, some talent, and then constant training made him a pro-footballer.

We all have our individual talents, our strengths and weaknesses. What makes us great is the constant use of those talents and skills. Constant training of those skills can make everyone a pro. Expecting to know everything and be great at everything is not the goal. It never was or shouldn't be.

We all have things we are better at than others, and there will always be things we are not even good at all. This makes us unique beings. This shouldn't make us feel any less but rather encourage us to show and live with our unique set of skills and talents. All together, we can enrich each other's lives, but so often we get judged, belittled, and rejected.

We are not made to be all the same, to be equally good at everything. We are all individuals with various interests and skills. So, let go of the belief of having to become someone or be someone in order to be good enough. You are already a masterpiece. You only have to realise it, and then live according to it.

This is where the concept of self-love comes in. Only if we love ourselves can we respect ourselves and live up to our own standards and values. Only then are we okay with expressing ourselves and not be scared to show our true nature and live the life we so desire.

Here are a few of the ways the lie of never being good enough can dominate our lives:

- When do you feel not good enough? This could be a particular environment when you are around particular people or in certain situations.
- When do you feel enough or good enough?
- What needs to happen specifically for you to feel not enough or not good enough?
- What are you doing specifically or what are you thinking when you feel good enough?
- What are you doing in your life in order to feel or be good enough? What are you doing in your work environment, in your relationships, etc.?
- Would you still be doing all of that work if you did feel good enough?

Once you accept and care for your instincts, live your humanness, uncover your inner drivers, transform your toxic monologue, and listen inward, then you finally will be able to see a vision of your life that will bring you not only healing but also a new motivator to come into your essence and live a life true to you. Only once you care for your needs and accept every part that makes you human will you feel safe within yourself. And only then will you be able to see the vision for your life that lies beyond fears and societal conditioning. This is the power of your root and crown chakra. It is basic. It is the fundament you build your life on and thus so important to heal first.

*If you did not have
any fear of rejection, what
would you do differently
in your life right now?*

Activate and balance your root chakra:

• Spend time in nature as often as possible. Nature helps with grounding and relaxation. Try to spend time in nature or with animals, ideally without any other form of distraction like a phone or work-related things. Aim to switch off and focus on the nature around you. Every day, aim to spend 30 minutes in nature and connect with the environment

• Move more. Sitting is poison for our bodies. When you are sitting long hours at a desk, aim to include breaks. Every 60 minutes, get up for at least 5 minutes and move. Climb the stairs. March in place using your arms. Complete 10 squats or 20 jumping jacks. Elevate your heart beat up to 110 per minute.

• Strength training is a great form of balancing your root chakra – especially strength training including your legs, buttocks and back. Connect to your body and humanness. Allows the root chakra to unload excess energy and create balance. It also helps to unload excess thinking energy around your head and channel it out through your legs to the ground. Energetic balance throughout the whole system.

• Get some 'light' food and aim to get as much natural sunlight as possible. Ideally, every morning go for a 20-minute walk outside. Even when it's cloudy the light is still strong enough to feed your cells. We are all light beings. This little activity is nurturing you and setting you up for the day.

• Bring your attention throughout the day back to your needs as a human being. Stop what you are doing and turn inward. Pay attention to your needs and follow them. Respect yourself.

• Pay attention to the quality of your sleep. During the night, your root chakra can let go of major stresses, and sleep is so important for body repair work and self-healing.

• Treat yourself throughout the day to some breaks. Give yourself a break from all the demands others have on you, but especially the demands you place on yourself. You are not an emotionless machine. You are a magnificent human being. Take time for yourself, and this could be meditating for 10 minutes, or just doing nothing and sitting in the sun. Schedule fun activities a few times a week and dedicate yourself to that particular activity i.e. gardening, meeting a friend for coffee, yoga, reading a book. Do this without thinking about anything else. Dedicate yourself to a moment of joy.

• Take time to eat. So often people tend to eat while working or doing something else. We nearly don't make time to celebrate the little moments where we nourish our body and mind with good food. Eating is a basic human need. Take conscious time to eat and enjoy the food. Feel how it does you good.

· Hectic lifestyles and unhealthy food choices tend to mess with our gut system. Our microbiome is interconnected with our root chakra. How can you reduce stress and change stress induced lifestyle choices? Support your gut health with a cleanse.

· Treat yourself to a foot and leg massage.

· Become friends with your fears and allow them into your heart. Make peace with them and take sessions with a coach or therapist to battle major fear issues that keep you from living the life you want to live.

· Healing foods: Ensure you eat sufficient protein in your diet. The more natural sources the better for your overall health and your root chakra. Foods like beans, pulses, nuts, soy products and tofu. Protein is important for our muscles, and they are a building block for our hormones. Getting sufficient protein is important for your body and health. Eat more root vegetables for a balanced root chakra like beetroot, potatoes, or carrots.

Activate and balance your crown chakra:

· Constantly question yourself, your opinions, your lifestyle and check in with yourself about how you could move out of your comfort zone.

· Do more crazy things, dedicate yourself to the experience of living with your inner genius and stop trying to have it all figured out.

· Let go of the need to control and have to understand everything, instead trust and have faith in others.

· Practice inversions – yoga poses help to change our perspectives and take us out of black-and-white thinking. Great poses are for example down dog or headstand.

· Unconditional self-acceptance of everything you are, including your little faults and differences. Practice self-forgiveness and self-love.

· Incorporate visualisation practices to your life, such as meditations, daydreaming, breathing exercises.

You can practice the following flows daily or whenever you feel like your root and crown chakra are out of balance. These are not fast-moving exercises but rather based on a more hatha yoga style. Meaning you get into the pose and while activating your muscles you focus on breathing deeply and becoming aware of how you feel in your body. Ideally you hold each pose for up to two minutes. You can also pick and choose just 3 or 4 poses you would like to do throughout the day instead of putting 30 minutes aside to do them all. Go with your inner knowing. Let your intuition guide you.

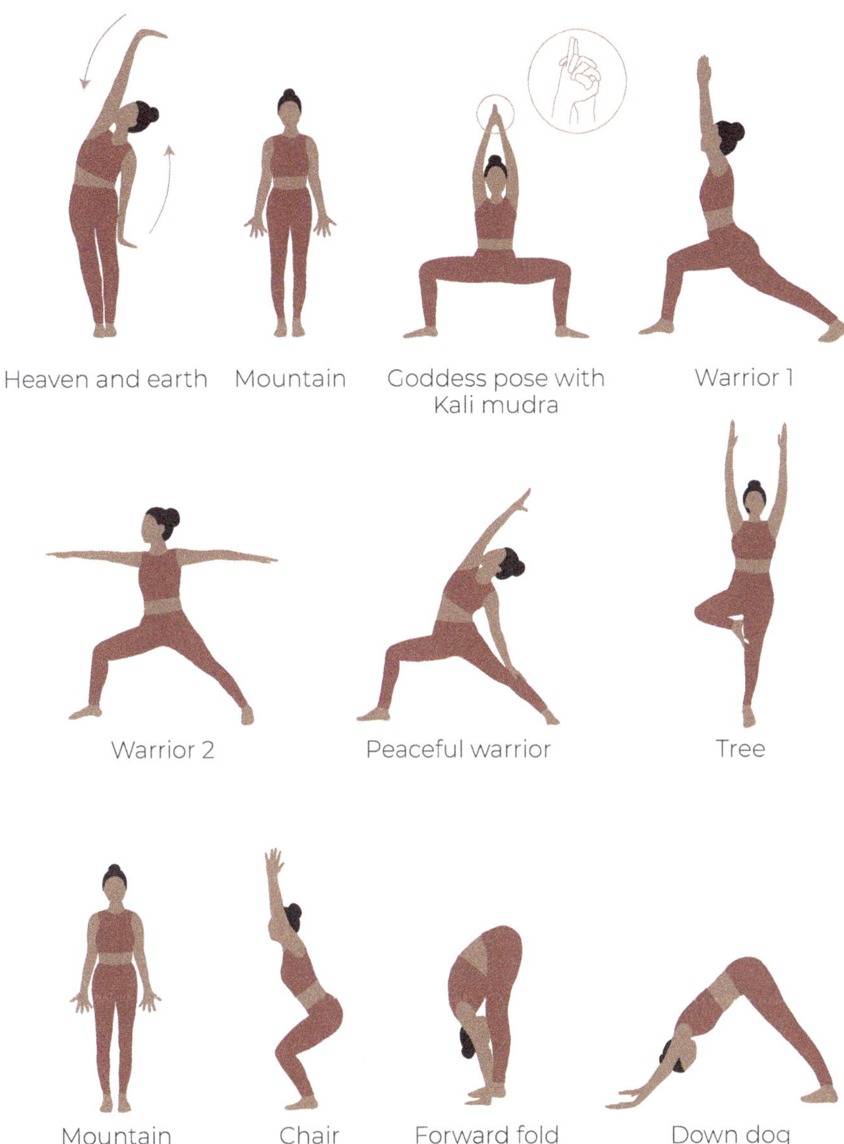

Heaven and earth
Mountain
Goddess pose with Kali mudra
Warrior 1
Warrior 2
Peaceful warrior
Tree
Mountain
Chair
Forward fold
Down dog

MEDITATION

This meditation is for finding stillness and should take five minutes. It helps us to breathe more fully and start the day with confidence and calmness. It is grounding and empowering.

Start in a standing position. Stand with your feet hip-with apart, spine lengthened upward, shoulders away from your ears, and head held high. Position your arms on your sides and let them hang relaxed.

Inhale and sweep your arms over your sides slowly up above your head until your hands are facing each other. Exhale slowly as you lower your arms in front of you, with your palms facing to the floor, and bring them back to your sides. Try to deepen and lengthen your breathing in accordance with the movement and try to feel the pause after each breath. Repeat this 15 – 20 times.

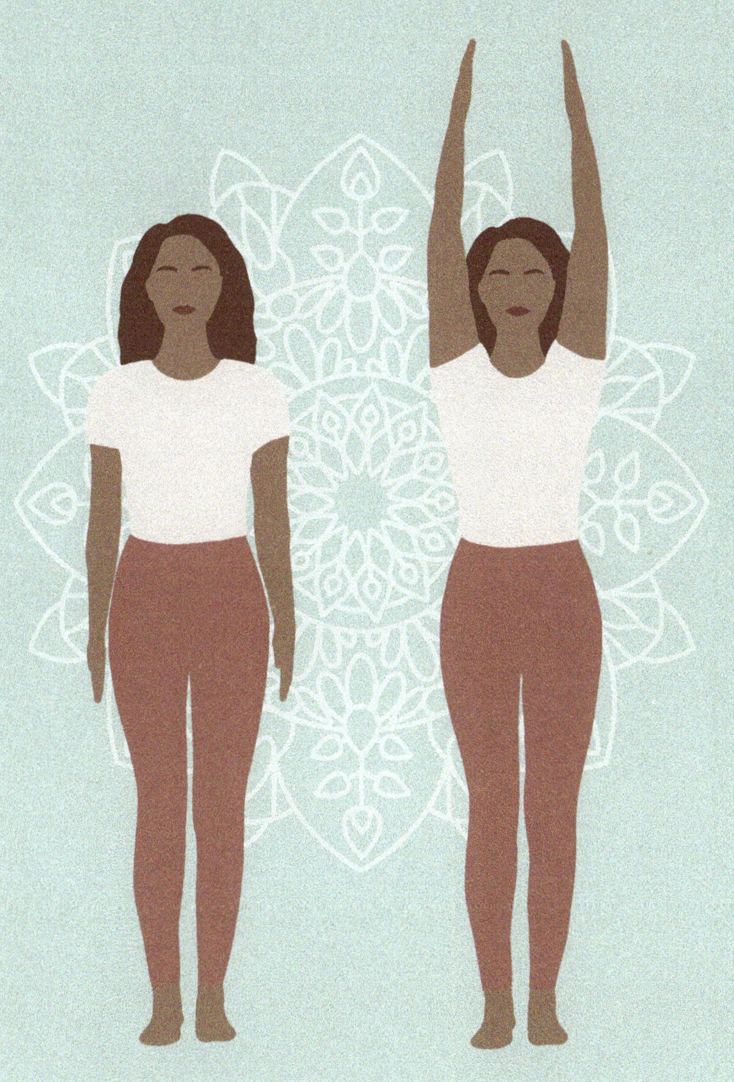

PART 3: BALANCE AND RECONNECTION

Can you feel your emotions fully? Do you remember what it feels like to be fully dedicated to something? Experience joy and pleasure to the full extent? Do you remember? Or has it been so long since you allowed yourself to feel...

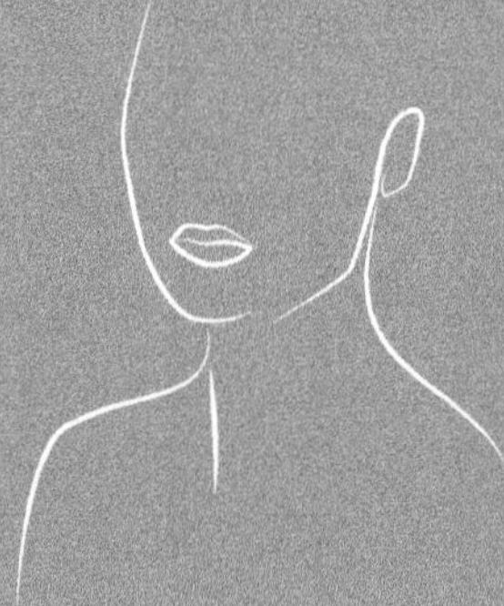

BODY AND MIND

Our bodies are pure magic. They constantly try to talk to us. They let us feel. However, when I was at my worst, I was focused on suppressing my whole spectrum of emotions.

As a kid in school, I was bullied because of my weight and my nationality. I learned that the rejection from others hurt. So, instead of getting hurt, I went numb. I acted as if it did not hurt me. I acted as if nothing could hurt me.

In my twenties, I was fully living inside my thick armour, not letting anything get to me, but I started to crumble under the enormous pressure that was building. How do I feel about someone or something? I couldn't tell. For years, my brain dictated what I should do, what I should be feeling, based on others around me. Let me give you two examples you might be able to relate to.

First, nutrition and body image. I really started to hate my body as a teenager. Being overweight was really bringing my self-worth down. So, I started to trial various diets. I started to exercise. When I eventually got to a healthy weight, that was no longer important. My mind and view on things mattered the most. My brain would still tell me I was not pretty enough. I thought that if I had a loving partner who would validate me, and tell me I was pretty enough, only then – I told myself – would I be happy.

There's no need for me to say that this is complete nonsense. The suppression of my feelings led to a distorted body image, which caused me to fall into a binge eating trap and enter a vicious cycle of self-hate. My body became my own personal battlefield.

I punished myself for not being how my mind told me I should be, and my mind was brain washed by magazines and what other people told me beauty looked like. I rejected myself on all levels and so I had a constant fight with my body until I hit burnout at age of 30.

To emphasise the power of our mind and its tricks, let's use a simple example of eating. When you eat, do you sometimes feel like a particular food is not good for you? Does your stomach feel sick, or could you pay more attention and hear your body rejecting the food? But does your brain try to tell you that it is healthy, or to continue eating it, whether it harms you or not?

This is a tiny example, but so many of us do this. Think of milk, think of a particular vegetable, think of junk food or sweets. For example, I cannot eat too much bread or foods that contain gluten. They might be great for others but for me it gives me feelings of being bloated and indigestion. Same goes with milk products, or junk food. If I eat them, my digestion is dead for days. Hence, our body knows better than our brain. Instead of following a particular diet, or letting our emotions dictate what to eat, we could gain a lot for our health from listening into our bodies.

I am not saying that our minds are useless, we need logic at times too. However, we live in a world where we think that the mind is the ruler of the body, and therefore key to all our success in life. Mind over matter. But without matter, there is no mind. We cannot live in favour of one over the other. We need to include the whole system. Our bodies, our hearts and emotions play a huge role in the whole system.

Another example was my marriage. It might have been love in the beginning, but over time it became more of a responsibility. I was married, I had to love my husband. At least, that's what I told myself. I had to take on the role of a wife and ensure that I pleased him, because that's what I believed growing up. That's what I told myself, that's what I had to do in order to receive the love I was so longing for. But was it true? No. But I couldn't tell what true love would feel like, or what the whole array of emotions would feel like, because the ruler was my mind. And with my mind as ruler, I was good at following the orders of my mind, and suppressing all those feelings that wanted to rise.

I existed in this area of conflict for years, between what my emotions wanted me to feel and what my head told me to do. I suppressed my emotions in order to be accepted and get the job done. I lived to please my partner, to make him happy. I lived according to my partner's values and dreams. His dreams became my dreams. His values became my values. His happiness became my highest goal. And so, I forgot about my needs, my feelings, and dreams.

Why did I do this? Well, back then I was clearly emotionally co-dependent. I was alone for a lot of my upbringing, my parents were immigrants and they both worked most of the time, so from a young age I learned that if I do what is expected of me, I will receive love.

So, I replicated this system of pleasing others in order to receive love in my relationship. All I wanted was to be loved, but instead of looking for this love inside myself, I gave my power away to the outside world. I was dependent on the validation of others to show me love or approve of me in order to feel good about myself. I would be disappointed when I didn't receive the acts of love I might have expected, but then suppressed any negativity or sadness. I would tell myself that's what I deserved. If I was lied to or emotionally abused, I would

still find a way to tell myself not to open up or speak my opinion, just to avoid a fight. I would forbid myself to feel hurt, and
I would just carry on with my day.

I would suppress my needs for a break from house chores,
and suppress my desires for a holiday or some nice treats for
myself at the expense of my partner. I even started to hate
myself for having a period because my partner didn't like it.
So, I rejected everything that was me, including the parts that
make me a woman. My cycle, my body, my feminine side.

Emotional suppression and emotional abuse in a co-dependent relationship can lead to self-hate and self-rejection. We
can tend to abuse ourselves through addictive behaviour like
drinking, excessive shopping, eating or not eating. I was at
war with myself, with my true self. I believed I was not worthy
of love. I believed I was not good enough to receive love. My
partner knew what he had to say or how he had to behave
so I would not listen to myself. To my inner whispers. And
soon the place I called home became my living hell. I was not
in love anymore. I woke up to the reality of having lived in a
cage, and that if I didn't break out from that cage soon, my
wings would be cut off and I wouldn't have a chance to flee.

I slowly started to accept that if I didn't speak up my truth,
that I was no longer in love, and allow my true feelings to
come through, my inner tension and suffering would never
end, and the cycle of self-rejection would lead my system

to crash. This constant fight between suppressing my emotions and leading with my head, where I told myself the most self-destructive lies, is exactly what pushed me to reach burnout on all levels: physically, mentally, emotionally, and energetically. A classic imbalance of your sacral and third eye chakra when suppressed or under constant stress. We suppress our emotions, which leads to stress and imbalance in the sacral chakra, which in turn impacts our third eye as it has to counterbalance, but gets under too much stress, leading to self-destructive thinking patterns. And the negative stress cycle continues.

This is where our body and mind are no longer working in sync and communication between them gets distorted. When you end up in burnout, your body and mind are exactly like this, no longer able to speak with each other. The whole system is out of balance, and it crashes.

TOPICS COVERED BY THE SACRAL AND THIRD EYE CHAKRAS

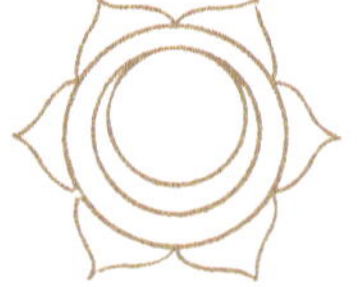

SACRAL CHAKRA

· Love for your own body, sexuality, and sensuality

· Love without control

· Joy of being yourself and dedicate yourself to your personal needs and being

· Creativity, playfulness, sense of adventure

· Vulnerability

· Allowing yourself to not know everything, to not have everything figured out, to let go of perfection

· Allowing yourself to feel all emotions and let them flow

· Love for beautiful things, flowers, and art

· Acceptance of your sexual desires and needs

· Having balance between directing your energy and letting go

· Setting healthy boundaries and saying no

· Taking responsibility for your own happiness

· Flexibility and adaptability

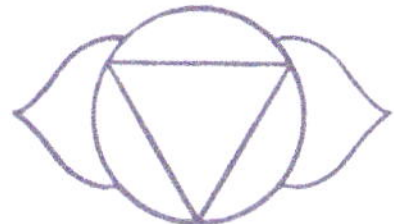

THIRD EYE CHAKRA

· Inner wisdom and intuition
· Power of thoughts, empowering as well as self-destructive (imbalance)
· Awareness of suppression techniques
· Development and awakening of psychic abilities
· Visions, vivid dreams
· Power of manifestation and visualisation
· Strong connection to pineal gland and thus to a field of unlimited opportunities
· Focus and attention
· Expansion of your consciousness and mental comfort zone
· Critical thinking and ability to see the bigger picture
· Going ways that seem impossible

POWER OF VULNERABILITY

We have learned to live according to the standards of others. We have learned what we are allowed to be and what not to be. Essentially, we have become scared of living life fully. We live according to the rules we have been told to live by, afraid of being our true selves and living the life we desire. We are afraid of expressing our truth. We have closed our hearts, learned to not listen to desires and true intentions, but to blindly follow the expectations of others.

Don Miguel Ruiz said it so nicely: "That is why humans resist life. To be alive is the biggest fear humans have. Death is not the biggest fear we have, our biggest fear is to take the risk to be alive – the risk to be alive and express what we really are. Just being ourselves is the biggest fear of humans."

We believe the lie that having a particular body, living a particular life, that having particular things is equal to status and social acceptance. By believing this, we close our hearts and hide the most vulnerable and important parts of ourselves. Being vulnerable has become something negative. Something bad. When in fact, it is a gift.

Rejecting ourselves because we believe we don't fit a particular image or that we don't follow the demands of others needs to stop. You must embrace the full being you are. Vulnerability means living with your heart wide open. Showing yourself as you truly are and not being afraid of not fitting in. Only then can we embrace life and ourselves.

Vulnerability means being open to new experiences and being open to live life! Being vulnerable is also accepting yourself for who you truly are. Once we decide to be vulnerable, we encourage others to do so, too. And thus, we attract also more and more like-minded people and help others to live with an open heart as well.

Ask yourself:
· What does it mean to you to be vulnerable?
· How would being vulnerable impact your life if you would allow yourself to be more vulnerable? What could happen?

Vulnerability is also about going with the flow. When we are constantly in touch with our feelings, when we no longer suppress them, we can then express a variety of feelings like anger, joy, sadness, love and others to the fullest. We accept all our emotions and thus are in flow with them which is much healthier for us overall.

This is when we are in the flow of who we are and what we feel. We are emotional beings, and we can express ourselves through emotions, which are basically our energy system – energy in motion. If we lock them away and hide our vulnerable parts, what we essentially do is kill our lifelines. If we would just stop judging our emotions and instead see them for what they are, we would be so much better off.

Yoga taught me that instead of saying "I am so angry", I should be saying "this is anger". This detaches myself from being the emotion, so that I observe that this emotion is currently present. Try this approach and see how it works for you. I have to admit I am not overly successful with it. However, for some this way of thinking helps them flow with their emotions. Something my spiritual coach taught me that works actually for some emotions so much better is to embrace the emotion. As with everything, emotions come and go. So when we own our emotion instead of constantly suppressing them or detaching ourselves from them, we can let them go even faster.

Only if you become an emotion, can you also decide to let that emotion go.

This is what it means to flow with them. If we don't, if we suppress negative feelings or parts of us that we deem inadequate, negative or that we are ashamed of, we literally poison our system and this leads to blockages in our energy system. Our energy gets depleted without being restored and life becomes dull and meaningless. Embrace and feel your emotions, and then let them go.

As you can see, vulnerability is so important because it allows us to no longer hide and suppress important parts of ourselves. We would no longer need our brain to be on alert and cut certain emotions out because we would no longer be afraid of feeling them. Feelings would come and go. We would allow ourselves to be human. We would accept ourselves with all our emotional spectrum. We no longer hide behind a mask of who we are not. We no longer fear emotions and, most importantly, they become our energy supplier instead of depleting our energy supplies.

The last point I would like to mention when it comes to vulnerability and living with your heart wide open is that once you allow yourself to be vulnerable you allow yourself to let go of things that do not suit you. You develop a compassionate outlook for yourself and others, which allows you to let go of negativity, of mistakes, of failures, of fear, and this is when healing can take place, because you finally allow wounds to heal without suppressing their pain and impact. This is true healing power at your fingertips.

RHYTHM OF LIFE

Whenever I had a tough time, someone around me would usually say, "Where there is rain, there will be also sun". There will bad times and there will be good times. This is part of life. The same principle is being used in traditional Chinese medicine. The concept of yin and yang. My Qigong teacher said we cannot live just in balance, because that would mean living in stillstand.

However, we should aim for reaching homeostasis. Homeostasis is a term from biology which describes the optimal functioning of our organism. Yin and yang are constantly aiming to balance each other out because sometimes particular emotions or stresses can impact our system.

Yin and yang energy is always in motion, it is never still, the one goes up and the other goes down, and vice versa. This is life. There are seasons. You might have heard that as the seasons pass, so do seasons of life. Winter usually is the time to rest, recover and sow the seeds. It needs darkness for the seed to develop and nurture in stillness. Then there is spring, where the seed inside you starts growing as everything else in nature does. In summer you are driving on your energy and actively creating your business success, your promotion and your relationships and projects. In autumn you harvest your successes. There are times of stillness and rest, there are times for action, and times for shining and times of darkness, but that doesn't mean something is good or bad. It is just the rhythm of life. Do you see the trees, flowers, or animals complain about the seasons or the weather? No. Because they learned to live with the rhythm of life.

If you can go with the rhythm of life, you win and save on a lot of stress and energy. If you go with the flow, it also means you have faith in life, and can rest assured that whatever comes your way will serve a purpose and will be for your highest good.

Because remember: life is always for you. Thus, we learn the skill of letting go. If we worked on our limiting beliefs and fears, when we have forgiven, and are finally able to go with the flow, then we also master the skill of letting go, because we know it is just temporary and whatever happened has lost its meaning the moment, we no longer attach to it. This is living in the now. Being present and actively giving life a chance to create the one we truly want to live.

SEXUALITY AND CREATIVITY

As you now know, our sacral chakra is also our sexual and creative centre. This means that if we ever had any trauma with sex or abuse it would cause an imbalance in this chakra. This also means that any illnesses of your sex organs could get dissolved with the energetic work on the sacral chakra. It is not only concerned with sexual intercourse, but also your sexual energy which relates to creativity. Creation of ideas and art. Dedication to the self and the flow of emotions as mentioned before. The balance of being and feeling through letting go.

For me, this was a tough topic. My body hate, rejecting my feminine energy and parts led me to have real issues in my late twenties with my period. My partner's disgust at my period made me learn to be disgusted by it too. My body rejected all sorts of additional hormones from my contraception, so I stopped taking the pill, and went for a non-hormonal solution. However, my cycle was still out of balance for one and a half years, and I had more days of being "on" than "off" my period. Only once I did the work on my sacral chakra, once I started loving and accepting myself and embracing my femininity, my whole cycle started to balance out. Learning to love and appreciate my body as it is now. Loving myself for who I am now. Saying 'no' to others and clearly setting boundaries so I can care for my needs made a huge difference to heal my distorted view on my femininity.

And so, my creativity began to flow. I never knew that I could be creative as I always suppressed that energy and side of me completely. My mind always told me I was not creative, I was analytical. But again, what does our mind truly know without our feelings and heart? I healed some past trauma when I found my true love. A partner who accepted me on all levels of my being, even embraced it, including my period. Experiencing this was what made me actually enjoy sex, come to embrace my period and fully unfold my creativity as a woman.

Issues like sexuality are difficult to resolve by ourselves. We need a loving partner who can support us, because through the experience with them we can heal and start seeing and feeling the truth. The truth of loving all of you because you are great just as you are. This is how healing can take place on this level. Sometimes we have to stand our ground for ourselves and let go of toxic relationships that harm us.

Finding balance between your emotions and thoughts and learning to flow is the key to healing your sacral and third eye chakra connection – your connection between body and mind. Once this connection is established and maintained your chances burning out ever again are reduced to zero.

WHERE YOUR FOCUS GOES, YOUR LOTUS GROWS

Let's not wait any longer. How can you tune in and actively manifest your dream life? Here are the main tools that have worked for many people, including myself. Just remember that in order to achieve successful and lasting change, changes need to be practiced daily. Repetition and consistency are key. Just thinking about something once a week is not enough to change your life. It needs constant dedicated practice and action. The following tools can assist you in tuning into the feelings and thoughts, the visions of how you want your life to be. Remember, focus and manifestation are part of your third eye chakra.

The way you feel literally dictates how your life goes. As much as you are what you think, trust me, you are just as much what you feel. You are an energetic being. Your body is made up of energy. Your cells are energy. Your organs are energy. If you struggle with this belief, let me explain that our ancestors and most Eastern traditions are based on energy. I am referring here to traditional Chinese medicine, Reiki Healing, Qigong, Yoga, Complementary health services like acupuncture, reflexology, energy healing and many more.

THREE VISION TOOLS

Vision board

The best tool to remind yourself every day about the greatness within you and show you how to manifest your dream life is to create a vision board and place it where you will see it often throughout the day. Create a vision board with everything you desire your life to be like. It is your VISION of your life. Tune into what you see. Imagine the feelings of having what you want and having achieved your dreams. Be grateful for already having what you want. Gratitude will accelerate your vision coming into existence. The two major forces that will help you in manifestation are love and gratitude so feel those two emotions from the bottom of your heart whenever you look at your vision board. Take a board or large A0 paper and pin or stick the images that represent the things you want to manifest. Write them all down. If you think I am old school and you want to do the same thing digitally, then create your vision board on your device and carry it with you every day. Use it as desktop background, print it out and display it all over your home. It is your vision. Your life. Happy creating!

Vision manifesto

Create your own vision manifesto. Your vision manifesto is based on your vision board, but it's where you
can summarise your dream life in words. Writing is
powerful. This manifesto is your vision declared in a
holy manner. Read it every morning and before going
to bed. Every time you feel low or when you're in a
bad mood, take this vision manifesto out and read it.
Make sure to write your vision manifesto in the present tense. As you are living it right now.

Meditation/ virtualisation

Meditation has the power to calm your system and
change your brain waves in order to let you enter
your subconsciousness. Bring in visualisation as part
of your meditation; and you can see things visually
in front of your inner eye. Add virtualisation, which is
the feeling of who you want to become, or the feeling
of what you will have if you achieve you desires, and
this way you can see and feel your vision come to life
during a meditation right in front of your inner eye.
Why is this so powerful?

Similar with changing your identity, imagining living your dream life, and being who you want to be in a meditation is like creating the neuronal pathways for this new reality to come forth. You live it first in your mind before it becomes real in your life.

Do this every morning when your subconscious mind is at its most receptive; you will not only set yourself up for a day in your best mindset, but you will train new beliefs for the feelings of experiencing what you wish for. This is how manifestation works. This is how you attract what you desire into your life.

THE POWER OF MANIFESTATION

The exercises above are great ways to bring harmony into your third eye chakra. However, I want to highlight what can cause imbalance in this chakra and explain how powerful it is. We are literally blind, as our third eye chakra can colour our view on how we see the world and it impacts our thoughts. It can literally put a filter on reality that makes us blind to our dreams and visions. We do not believe that something better is possible for us, nor do we believe in our own greatness. We get comfortable believing what others tell us and stop believing in our dreams and stop creating our own thoughts. We stop using our own mind to make our own opinions. We are influenced by media and social media which shape our world view, our opinions on life and on ourselves. We stop thinking for ourselves. We struggle to bring our creativity to life; we lose the creative genius within us.

This is the danger when we let our third eye get distorted energy-wise. Now you can also see the link even more to our creative centre – our sacral chakra. We need them both to work together in balance in order to unfold our full potential.

The third eye chakra is our manifestation centre; it is our sending and receiving antenna. We can send focused energy into the universe and so attract what we desire. We receive what we long for if the energy frequency is matching. However, for this to happen we need to allow life to inspire us.

We need to be in flow with who we are and our emotions.

Any emotional suppression leads to distortion in our third eye chakra. And as mentioned before, when our third eye is imbalanced, we tend to think negative thoughts and doubt our greatness. This can happen when we feel like what we do in life is meaningless. For example, a meaningless job or relationship. This is when our third eye chakra becomes stressed. It produces thoughts that are self-destructive and not beneficial for us. However, if we allow ourselves to think big and do the things that give us meaning, this is when we will have it easier to live a happy and healthy life, as our antennas for manifestation are set up for our highest good. Again, this is where we need the balance of our sacral and third eye chakra as we take our creative force to actually create and do the things that give us meaning.

By now you might have come to understand the link between those two chakras especially when it comes to manifestation. I would like to introduce a concept created by David Hawkins, who identified the vibration we humans emit when feeling various emotions. The chart on the next page gives you a nice overview. The more negative the emotion you feel, the lower your frequency. The more positive the emotion, the higher the frequency.

It is important to highlight that we all have a particular go-to emotion which we feel the most throughout the day. During my crisis, it was mostly a mix of fear, desire and anger. There were times where I got frustrated and angry at everyone and everything. However, this was also the time of my life that led me to burnout. With those emotions in the driving seat, I was not only sending out low vibrational energy but also attracting events, circumstances and people with exactly that kind of frequency back into my life. And there I would be, sitting in this cycle and wondering why life was such a pain. However, after becoming aware of our energy system and of how we can turn things around, I am now mostly in the range of acceptance, reason and love – which literally allows me to live a completely different sort of life. Right now, the world is experiencing an astronomical level of fear, and as such it is vibrating very low. This also explains the situation on Earth and why so many events are happening that magnify the feeling of fear.

I hope that reading this book helps your healing journey and allows you to rise to your true self and raise your vibration. Because your rise will contribute to the overall rise of the world consciousness.

EMOTIONAL SCALE OF EMPOWERMENT

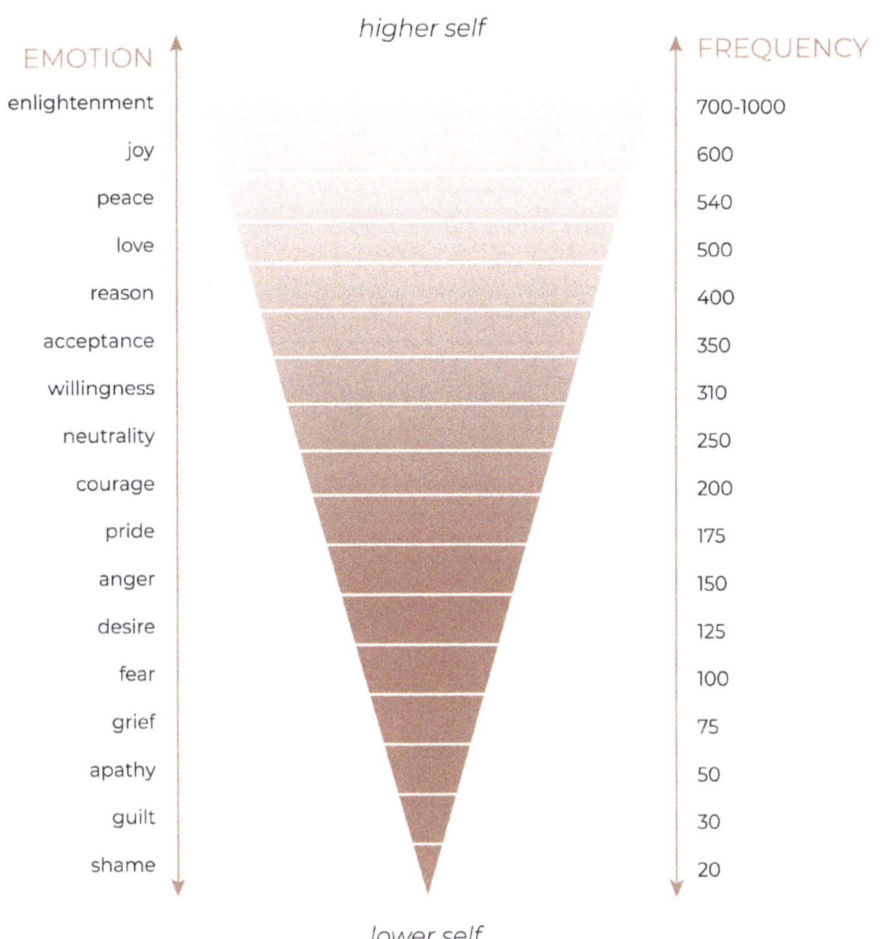

How would it feel like to be who you truly want to be? What would this version of you think, feel and do? What can you do to feel and think like this version of you now?

Activate and balance your sacral chakra:

· Connect with the element of water. Observe the water in rivers, lakes, and in the sea. Take a bath or actively enjoy your shower. Drink plenty of fresh water daily.

· Massage your belly. Massage yourself but also any other form of massage is a great way to balance and activate your sacral chakra, any other acts that help you to feel your body.

· Practice forgiveness and compassion, especially towards your father figure.

· Allow yourself to be vulnerable, show your emotions and let them come and go. Stop suppressing them or being ashamed of them.

· Take responsibility for your feelings and emotions. Stop blaming others for the way you feel and step up and make your life independent from other opinions and feelings.

· Set boundaries and say "no" in order to nurture yourself and care for your own needs, end the 'dis-ease to please'. Ask yourself how you can practice this more.

· Become aware of the things that make you happy and find time to follow your needs and care for yourself. Don't expect others to do that for you.

· Become aware of your sexuality and your personal sexual needs and find ways to explore and live them. Suppressing those feelings leads to further blockages and can lead to forms of addiction to food, drugs, and alcohol. It is not only the act of intercourse, but also exercising your sexual energy. It is the mother of your creativity that wants to be explored and lived. Live your creative genius.

· Practice flexibility and adaptability. Stop planning everything strictly or getting upset if things don't go the way you want them to. Life can't be planned. Life is to be lived and you adapt when required. Stay flexible, and stay open to change. Embrace it, don't fear it. Let life surprise you.

· Consume healing foods: naturally sweet foods like fruits – particularly orange in colour like oranges, apricots, mangoes, sweet potatoes and peaches. Consume hormone building seeds to your meals like flaxseed, pumpkin seeds and sesame seeds. Most importantly, don't go on a drastic, depriving diet, this harms you psychologically and will impact your thyroid. Practice intuitive eating and aim to eat as many natural foods as possible.

Activate and balance your third eye chakra:

· Participate in regular meditation practice.

· Create your life's vision. Start dreaming big, create a vision board, use your imagination to create the life you want to live, and allow yourself to believe that something more than what you are living right now is possible.

· Limit the information flow from the news, social media, and the media overall, and find some inspiration from within. Listen inwardly and become aware of your inner wisdom. Read books that inspire you.

· Massage or lightly tap the point between your eyebrows to gently activate your third eye.

· Ask yourself questions. When you do not know the answer, let your intuition provide it for you. This practices your ability to listen inward and stops you depending on your critical brain only.

· When particular thoughts come up, like blame and negative self-talk, pause and ask yourself where they are coming from. Sometimes we are so used to self-destructive thinking patterns that we do not even notice that these are actually not our own thoughts, but a belief that was planted in us when we were young. It is time to interrupt such thinking patterns.

· Write down the top five negative beliefs you have about yourself and re-write them into your top five inspiring affirmations. You can use them as your password, write them on post-its and pin them where you can see them often. You can read them every morning as a reminder of your greatness. Save them in your phone and you can read them every time you go to the toilet.

· Take in light food. As with the root chakra, light can impact and empower our energy and DNA healing, but also activate our pineal gland. Aim to get as much natural sunlight as possible. Ideally, every morning you should go for a 20-minute walk outside. Even when it's cloudy, the light is still strong enough to feed your cells. We are all light beings. When you breathe, imagine your breath lighting up your brain centre behind your eyes, where your pineal gland is located and visualise how it is being illuminated with every breath you take in.

· The more you start living and embracing the true self, the more balance you will create in your third eye chakra.

· Take in healing foods, especially purple foods like kale, blueberries, grapes, aubergine and cabbage, or any other purple food you may find. Add some herbs that enhance the brain function to your foods like ashwagandha and bacopa, but also nuts like walnuts and Brazil nuts.

HEALING INTERVENTIONS

YOGA EXERCISES

As with the previous yoga poses you can choose to use them as a gentle flow or as Hatha yoga sequences. Do the moving poses for a total of 10 breaths in and out and hold the static poses for up to two minutes or longer.

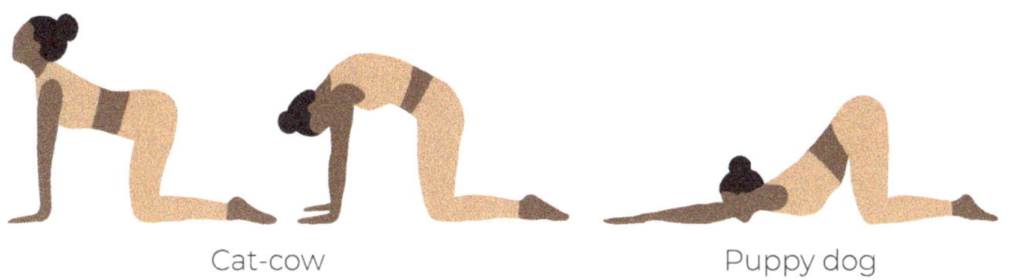

Cat-cow   Puppy dog

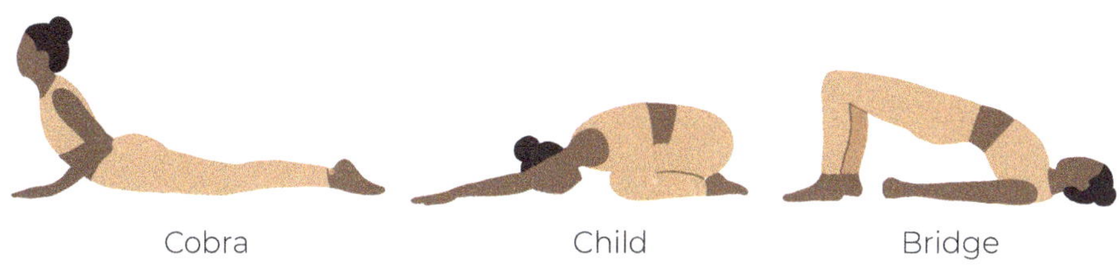

Cobra   Child   Bridge

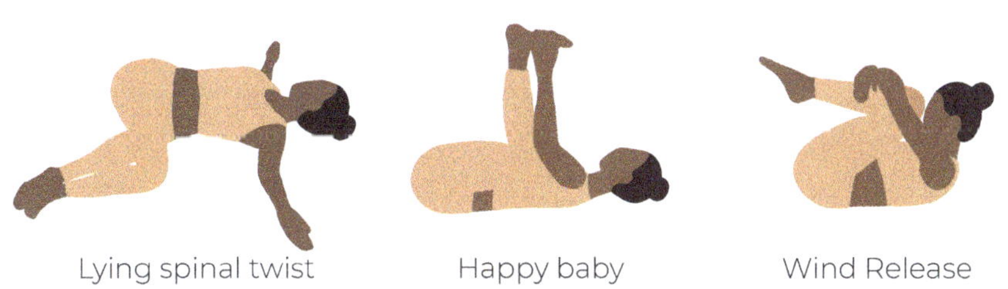

Lying spinal twist   Happy baby   Wind Release

MEDITATION

Nadi Shodana (nostril breathing), is great for emotional balance and balancing both brain halves.

When stressed, our brains are all over the place. Therefore, it helps to balance the energy between both sides of the brain to reduce stress and find inner calm, while stabilizing our emotions.

Sit in a comfortable position. For this exercise, use either hand. Let's use for this example the right hand. Bend your index and middle finger. Take one deep breath in and out. Then press your right thumb on your right nostril and breathe in through your left nostril for four counts. Hold your breath and count to four.
Then press your right ring finger on your left nostril and breathe out through your right nostril for four. Then breath in through the right nostril for four counts. Hold the breath again for a total count of four before moving your thumb back on your right nostril; so you breathe out for four counts through your left nostril. Breathe in through the left nostril. Hold for four counts. Press the right ring finger again on the left nostril and repeat for a round of twelve times or even longer. Then take a break by taking three deep breaths in and out.

Repeat Nadi Shodana for two more rounds.

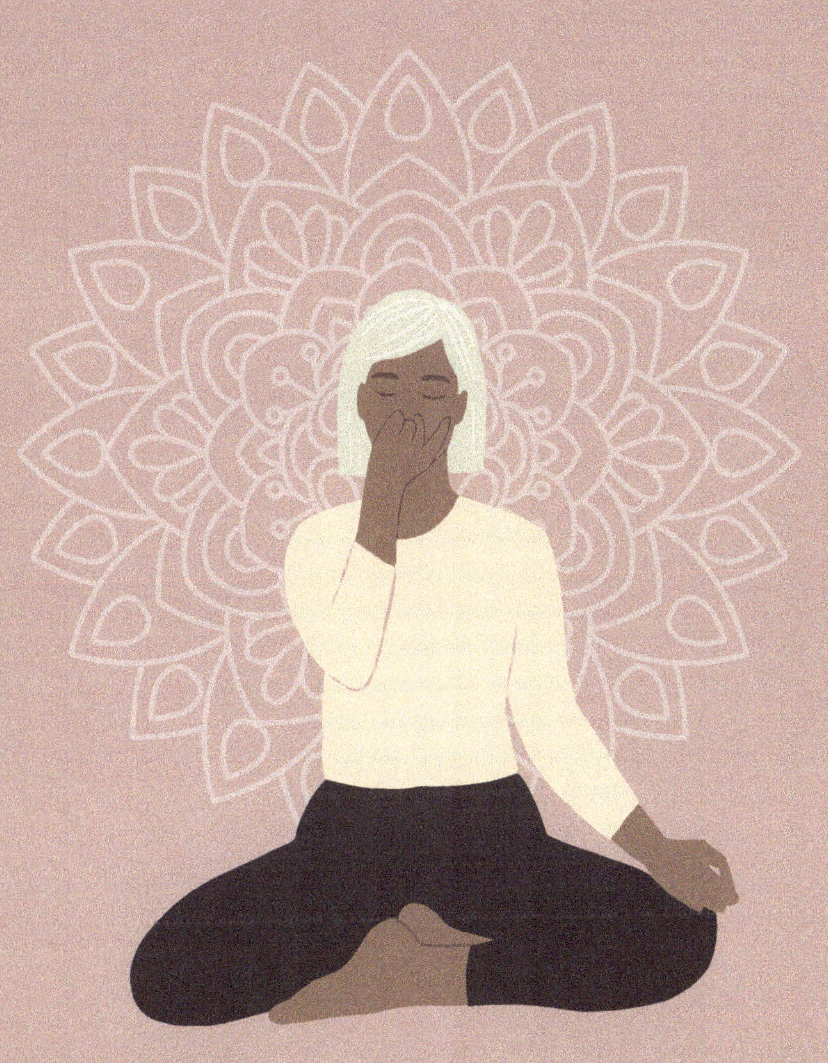

PART 4:
YOUR UNIQUE AND PERSONAL POWER

If you could say something to this world, what would you have to say right now?

CAN YOU BE INTENSE, POWERFUL, AND HONEST WITH YOURSELF?

Moments of complete frustration and anger. Times when you notice that everybody and everything around doesn't make sense. When you get angry at the government, the weather and your finances. When you waste all your energy and time on things and people that do not actually matter and do not add any value to your life or yourself.

How often were you in such moments and places? The Covid pandemic is a classic example. We channelled a lot of energy into something, and in doing so, achieved nothing. We blamed others, we got angry. But really, what did it change?

Your solar plexus chakra is your power source. It brings you energy. Your personal power. It is linked closely to your throat chakra because, in order to exercise your will power, you have to communicate your thoughts and opinions, don't you? And that is exactly where your throat chakra comes in. It is your communication centre, and also the centre of creation and identity. While your sacral chakra together with your third eye bring ideas to life in your mind, you need the solar plexus energy and your throat chakra to literally birth them into the world so they can take shape and can be shared.

You might know people who are very shy and don't speak up for themselves. They are easily dominated by others because they don't step into their power, but now you know living life fully means stepping into your power.

Your self-worth goes down the toilet when you give your power away. This is where you compare yourself with others, when you are not willing to accept and see your uniqueness. Accepting that you can be different, and this is okay. It is actually a great thing. If we don't believe that we are unique and special, we believe we are replaceable, that we are disposable. Living your life constantly comparing yourself to others seems like madness now, doesn't it? It seems like living a lie.

Lies are toxic to your solar and throat chakra. Not only when lying to others, but especially when lying to yourself. I can't even remember how often I lied to myself. Telling myself lies made me feel better, or feel nothing at all. I ignored my truth because the truth might hurt me or remind me to step into my power, where I lacked the courage to do so. But in doing this, I was blocking my throat chakra to express myself. And letting my solar plexus chakra get stressed and use energy against myself instead of for myself. The problem we have is that we are so used to lying to ourselves that we do not even notice it.

Speaking my truth was what set me free. Two examples I would love to share are about the co-dependent relationships I had with my parents and my partner. Since I was a child, I've always felt responsible for my parents. So, no matter what decision I was to take in my life, I always made them dependent on my parents. Would they be okay with it? I always sought their blessing or approval. I might still have done things they disagreed with, but their disagreement would make me not enjoy what I was doing because I knew they were not happy.

When I hit burnout last year, my therapist noticed this co-dependent relationship to my parents and, as a result, I sat down with them and had an honest conversation. I said I was sorry, but I could no longer be responsible for their happiness. When I wanted to go and live and work abroad for a bit, they obviously wanted me to stay but I needed to follow my calling for my own good. It was important to ensure they were responsible for their own happiness, and that I, as their child, would always be there for them, but the only responsibility I have now is to myself, my happiness and my life. This was not an easy conversation, but it was so freeing, and it helped me heal parts inside me that were deeply hidden.

With my ex-husband, it was becoming clear that we were no longer a match and didn't fit together. I tried to tell myself it would get better, just work for it, but the truth was simply: no, it wouldn't. Because there was no love anymore. The conversation was painful because I knew in his world it all made still sense. However, I had to speak my truth and that was that I could no longer continue, and I wanted a divorce. It was one of the most painful and uncomfortable moments I had thus far in my life, but at the same time it was the most liberating moment I have ever experienced. I spoke my truth, stayed true to my true self, and took my power over my life back.

The point I try to make is that we are responsible for our life. You are in charge. End of story.

We so often tend to give the responsibility of our life away to others. May it be our boss, our parents, neighbour or our pet. But what we are essentially doing is not living our power. Not living our life.

And this chapter is all about taking this power back so you can live the life you want to live. This is the action part.

TOPICS COVERED BY THE SOLAR PLEXUS AND THROAT CHAKRA

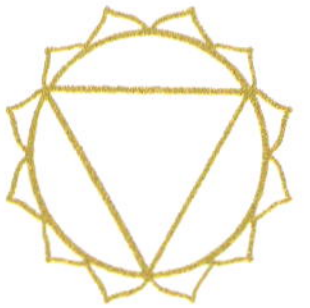

SOLAR PLEXUS CHAKRA

· Courage to go your own way and follow your interests.

· Balancing your inner needs with the outside demands.

· Healthy distancing to the environment and other people's business.

· Self-worth independently from achievements and material success.

· Having a powerful self-image.

· Healthy management of money and time.

· Immunity towards judgements, you don't take things personally.

· Personal power and setting boundaries.

· Being consequent and staying true to yourself, not giving in once you expressed your truth just to please others and feel better. Especially, in the beginning once you start taking a stand for yourself it might feel horrible as for so long pleasing others was your norm. But it will get better and you will feel better each time you stay true to yourself.

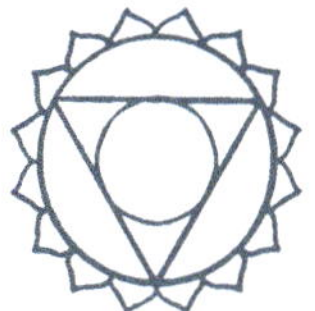

THROAT CHAKRA

- Communication with yourself and others.
- Self-expression of your needs, dreams and wishes.
- Living your talents and exploring them.
- Creating space and time for your own personal needs.
- Being authentic and true to yourself.
- Heal your fear of rejection.
- Taking responsibility for your own life, happiness and health and stopping the blame game.
- Realising your own uniqueness and importance in this world.

THE POWER OF CHOICE

To demonstrate the interconnectedness between the chakras again, if we suppress our emotions (sacral chakra) constantly, then it can lead to emotional instability, which can in turn lead to an anger explosion or sudden unexplained crying. So, you might suppress them in your sacral chakra, however the solar plexus chakra is the one that leads to the explosion of a single emotion and feelings of helplessness. Feelings of helplessness are a sign that our solar plexus is out of balance. We are not living in our personal power – a major area for the solar plexus chakra. We then struggle to express ourselves (throat chakra) which hits our self-worth, this in turn kickstarts our negative self-talk (third eye chakra). It continues until we give into feelings of fear that drive us relentlessly to please others, which then turns to neglecting our own human needs which brings imbalance into the root chakra which obviously impacts our crown chakra. And so, the vicious cycle continues. But how do we achieve balance? By becoming aware of the power of choice.

Many of us believe that we do not have any power or choice, but the truth is we do. For example, you do not have to go to work. I mean, nobody is putting a gun to your head, threatening to kill you if you don't go. There might be factors (inner drivers) that push us to go to work, things like paying the bills, maintaining our social status etc. But you have a wide spectrum of choice available to you.

You decide what kind of job you do, what sort of people you want to spend your time with. You decide if you want to participate in negativity, when instead you can choose to disconnect from the news and social media and surround yourself with people who do you good. The true essence of our solar plexus chakra is to gain power back over ourselves and our lives. Be open to whatever happens around you, but still be able to differentiate between what has value in your life and what does not. What is just noise, and has no further impact on your wellbeing? Yes, you can get upset at the laws in place, at the government, the weather, why Jane got a promotion and you didn't, why your sister is a better dancer – but what does it really matter to your life? What does getting upset and obsessed with these factors do to your life? Does it make you feel better? Are you happier when you get upset? Are you gaining anything from it?

Decide what you want and what is important to you. Don't get involved in stuff that doesn't concern you. This is the first step in taking your personal power back. Stop wasting energy on stuff that is pointless and outside of your influence. Focus your energy on yourself and the things you can actually have an impact on now.

Another form of choice is choosing to be immune to the judgement of others. How often do you take things personally?

Say you buy a new dress. Someone might say "Oh, what a beautiful dress!" and that makes you feel good, because you received validation. However, two hours later, someone else might say "Oh, the colour is weird." and there goes your confidence, trickling down the drain, because it is a form of negative judgement. Because one person doesn't like the colour, all of a sudden you feel your self-worth lessen, and you can't wait to go home and take it off.

Once we stop taking judgement personally and accept that everyone is entitled to their own opinion, to their own belief system and way of life, this is when we reach a new level of freedom. Let's be honest, there are over seven billion people living on this planet, so we cannot be all the same and think alike. Every single one of us has a unique way of looking at this world. A unique way of doing things.

Instead of seeking conformity, embrace your individual signature and contribution to this world. Stop judging others who do things differently and stop taking judgement from others personally. When you understand that we are all unique and do and see things differently, then you can accept this reality and develop a level of understanding and acceptance that leads to inner peace and balance.

When you reach this understanding, you will not hate others because they are "better", or because they do things in a totally different way, one that you are unable to comprehend.

Instead, you will have compassion and accept their differences. You will stop comparing yourself to others. Rather than zooming in on your short comings, you will see something in another person that calls for your own greatness to come forth. Because whatever it is you see in the other person that you admire, you can only notice it because it is already a part of you. You just need to start living it.

So often people compare themselves and end up frustrated, believing they will never be as good, or pretty or successful as other people are. But this way of thinking is literally giving their power away. Self-sabotaging their potential and progress without even trying. Instead of seeing other people who are more successful, prettier, and better as a motivation to become better themselves, they see them as confirmation of their own inability.

Whichever way you want to look at it, it always comes down to your own choice – and this is where your true power lies, where you can achieve personal freedom and evolution.

Who do you want to be? What do you have to start believing and doing in order to be who you truly want to be?

PERSONAL POWER

Power is an important and difficult topic, and for this reason I would like to go one step further to talk about it.

When we talk about power it can sometimes leave a bitter taste, like we are using someone for something. I had this feeling in the beginning as well. However, I think most people who do not exercise their own power might think this way, and I certainly was one of those people who lived to please others and give my personal power rather away instead of using it to stand up for myself and do the things that do my mind, body and soul good. Growing up we are told to be polite, be good to others, which are all valid points, but to what expense is that okay? Ask yourself the following questions and become aware of how you are dealing with power in your life:

- How do you feel about the word 'power'?
- When throughout your day do you feel powerful?
- What needs to happen for you in order to feel powerful?

Now think about the opposite:

- When during the day do you feel powerless?
- What needs to happen for you to feel powerless?
- What were you told about power when you were growing up? What did you learn from others about being powerful or

powerless? Were you told that one thing can be better than the other? Did you learn something in particular about being powerful or powerless?

- Do you fear to losing people if you would take your power over your life back?
- What can you do in order to take your power back?

You are powerful.

You are powerful because the only one who can change and navigate your life is you. Only you have that power over what you want to do and what you can do. However, if you choose to give your power away then, of course, it must feel like you don't have any power at all.

Another big misconception is that people believe we need to constantly fight for what we want. Sometimes we have to fight and still don't get what we desire, but sometimes the reason for that is simply that we don't live aligned with our heart. If you follow other expectations instead of your own, then the things you desire will not come to you. Life is actually always for us. Life wants us to live actively and experience its magic. But we are so influenced by others and the society and opinions that we don't dare to think bigger than we can. Don't dare to do more than we can or do what we truly desire to do.

If we live on autopilot, we don't even believe that there are other options available to us than the life we live at that moment. If you end up in a place where you feel unwell then that is a sign to change something – either about yourself or about your surroundings. Maybe this is the perfect time for some introspection. Become aware of the things in your life you no longer want to have, to deal with, to experience, or to be treated like and assess what needs to change in your life areas of career, self-care, partnership, sex, family, friends, health, finances, adventure and fun.

Once you are aware of what you no longer want in your life, you can start making changes. Stop allowing things that no longer serve you to be in your life.

THE BIGGEST LIE WE TELL OURSELVES

If I ask you, "How are you?" what would be your answer? May, I guess?

Your answer might be: "I am fine."

But your job exhausts you, your partnership annoys you, your stress levels are through the roof. What are you telling yourself after a bit of a rant?

"I am fine. Let's continue this madness."

When the question arises and begs for change, what is your answer? Are you willing to make the major changes in order to end your suffering? Set boundaries? May I take another guess?

Your answer might be "I can't do it. I have to continue. It is okay."

We tell ourselves we are fine when we are not. We tell ourselves that change is hard, that we can't do what we truly desire. We would disappoint others. They might not approve, and we lack the strength to stand our ground.
.
So, what are we doing instead? We keep lying and pretending to ourselves. Have you ever wondered what is worse, to lie to

someone else, or to lie yourself? I am not sure about you, but I never asked myself that question until recently. I was taught to always speak the truth and not to lie to others, but what I also learned along the way was keep lying to myself. Letting myself down on every occasion.

The truth is – since we are talking honestly – that embarking on change or doing something like following our heart is not something we cannot do. We can do it. We really can. The only thing we fear is rejection, and failure. The fear of what others think of us if we do what we truly desire in our heart to do. Change would be easy if we didn't depend on the opinions of others to dictate our worth.

Do you remember a time of change? A time when you were ready to go, but the resistance around you was the thing that made you stop? My friend, after 10 years of marriage, wanted a divorce. She never spoke much about what happened during those ten years, but things were bad and ugly things had happened. After three years of self-torture, she finally acted. It took all her courage, but she told her husband that she wanted a divorce, that there was no love anymore and she couldn't stand pretending that there was something left to give. She wanted it to end.

I must say, I could relate. I told her the best thing she could do was to follow her heart and do what was right for her. But what was shocking was the resistance of her so-called 'best friends', and even her mother. They told her she was making a horrible mistake. That she would not be able to sustain herself, or pay for bills. I was shocked how little they knew my friend, because she was more than capable of doing all of that and so much more.

But what this story shows you is that change would be so much easier if everybody cheered us on for doing it. However, this is wishful thinking. If we would allow ourselves to be truly independent and, for once, be honest with ourselves, we would be capable of so much more. If we would finally allow our sleeping potential to rise and live a heart-led life filled with joy, health and excitement.

Another important aspect is self-expression and speaking your truth. I barely spoke my truth in my teens or twenties. I must have done so as a child, by doing things like crying and getting upset when I felt like it. So did you. But the authentic me only came out around the age of thirty. Before I was suffocating my authentic voice and creativity. Constantly suppressing them just to be part of the masses, too scared of my own light coming out and shining. I did not believe in my own self-worth.

Your throat chakra is linked to your thyroid. An imbalance there can cause your thyroid stress. As you know by now, when I reached burnout, I had been giving my personal power away. Pleasing others non-stop. Loosing myself. Barely speaking my truth and lying to myself so often I couldn't even count how many times I did.

This deception leads to a disruption of our internal communication, where our head goes against our body. When I was twenty, I developed an underactive thyroid. Throughout that decade, life was not fun at all, and my daily dose increased until it reached 175µm by the age of 27. To give you a bit of an indication, once diagnosed with an underactive thyroid you usually start with 25µm and depending how it goes you might just increase the dose a little over the years. I reached nearly the maximum possible dose, although from the scans my thyroid looked perfectly healthy but not my blood results. Doctors told me I would have to take pills for the rest of my life. The only hope I got was from a traditional Chinese medicine (TCM) practitioner, who told me that with energy healing, personal development and healthy lifestyle I could get my thyroid in check, and hopefully get off the meds completely. And I did.

I believe there are other factors that play into how and why we lie to ourselves. How often do we try to be polite to avoid upsetting or hurting others? How often do we blame others instead of taking responsibility? How often do we expect others to know what is going on with us without communicating our needs? We need to stop blaming the universe, the constellations, the weather or that other person for our misery. Take responsibility for our own life and stop lying to yourself.

SUCCESS IS PERSONAL

What is success? The Cambridge Dictionary (2021) defines success as: *"the achieving of the results wanted or hoped for"* or *"something that achieves positive results."*

Do you define success like this? Most people define success as something materialistic, like living in a big house, driving a fancy car, wearing branded clothes, travelling to luxury resorts, or having a particular job. But, don't you agree, this is something that society sees as success?

I believe success is very personal.

Success is something that comes from intention and focus.

If you set your intention on your goal and focus on it and do everything that needs to be done in order for you to achieve that goal, you will. As long as it is important to you, and it is your goal, you will push to achieve it. Success has different meanings for different people. For some, it means being happy and healthy, for others it means wealth. Let me ask you, what does success mean and feel like for you? When you close your eyes and think about it, what does success really mean to you? How does success really feel to you?

YOUR VALUES

Our values are so important when it comes to making life choices. Sometimes we are coasting, and of course sometimes we make decision that come back to bite us in the behind. So, why are values so important? You've just created your unique definition of what success means to you, and you've constructed your vision manifesto. You have an idea what you no longer want in your life.

Values are like foundations, or pillars, that ensure your dream house stays stable and is built the way you want it to be built. Values help you enormously to stay true to yourself, to stay on track of achieving your goals, and serve as your inner compass so you never get lost. Metaphorically, we can say your heart is your value navigation system. It gives you feelings about what is right and wrong. Then it is our mind that decides what is right or wrong. Not everybody can immediately establish a heart connection (this takes time and practice), and therefore values can serve just as well instead. Now, if you are still recovering from burnout, have recently come out of it, or you live an incredibly stressful life, a heart connection might take a little while to establish. You might struggle to trust it at first. Therefore, values are a great navigation tool to have. So, let's have a look what your values are.

From the list below, mark all the words that resonate with you. Then, narrow down your top ten values if you can. Bring your top values down to your top five. What are they? If they are not part of the list, please write those down that come to your mind that feel right for you. Once you have established your top five core values reflect on them for a bit.

Abundance

Acceptance

Accomplished

Achievement

Acknowledgement

Activeness

Adaptability

Adoration

Adventure

Affection

Agility

Alertness

Ambition

Amusement

Anticipation

Appreciation

Attractiveness

Availability

Awareness

Balance

Beauty

Belonging

Benevolence

Bliss

Boldness

Bravery

Brilliance

Calmness

Capability

Care

Carefulness

Celebrity

Certainty

Challenge

Charity

Charm

Cheerful

Clarity

Cleanliness

Clear minded

Cleverness

Comfort

Commitment

Compassion

Confidence

Congruency

Connection

Directness

Discipline

Discovery

Discretion

Diversity

Dominance

Dreaming

Drive

Education

Effectiveness

Efficiency

Elegance

Empathy

Encouragement

Endurance

Energy

Enjoyment

Entertainment

Enthusiasm

Excellence

Excitement

Experience

Expertise

Extravagance

Extroversion

Fairness

Faith

Fame

Family
Fashion
Fearlessness
Fidelity
Fierceness
Financial
Fitness
Flexibility
Flow
Fluency
Focus
Freedom
Friendliness
Fun
Gentility
Giving
Grace
Gratitude
Growth
Happiness
Harmony
Health
Heart
Helpfulness
Honesty

Hospitality
Humility
Humour
Imagination
Impact
Impartiality
Independence
Inspiration
Integrity
Intelligence
Intimacy
Intuition
Joy
Leadership
Learning
Liberty
Logic
Love
Majesty
Mindfulness
Motivation
Mysteriousness
Openness
Optimism
Passion

Peace
Sacredness
Satisfaction
Security
Seductive
Self-control
Selfless
Sensitive
Sexy
Sharing
Shrewdness
Significance
Spirit
Spirituality
Stability
Teamwork
Thankful
Thorough
Thoughtful
Traditional
Tranquillity
Trust
Trustworthy
Truth
Uniqueness

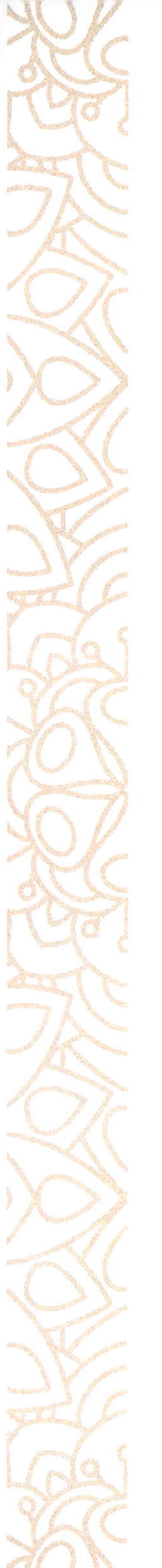

REFLECTION MOMENT

When do you know you are living your values?

What would you have to do or change for you to be able to live up to your values?

Where in your life are you currently living up to them and where not?

What are actions steps you can take in the life areas where you don't live up to them?

STOP ASKING FOR PERMISSION

You are creating a life for you. The things you do are meant to help you achieve the things you want to have and create. You do everything for your wellbeing and yourself, not for anybody else.

This means that you don't need approval, permission or any other form of acceptance from anybody but yourself. If it feels right for you, then trust it. On your way to living your best life and following your bliss there will be more than enough people who don't understand what you are doing – and that's often the case for our family members. They just don't understand what you are doing and how you can earn a living from your passion, or how you choose not to follow societal norms. But that is their problem. Not yours.

You don't have to persuade them either. They will most likely come around once they see you succeed and see your happiness. But until then, don't waste your valuable time on trying to persuade others to get their stamp of approval. And don't waste your time on self-doubt either. You are meant to live a magnificent life and trust me when I say that it sometimes sounds easier than it is, but that's only because you are doing it, for the first time, listening and seeking what your heart desires you to do.

Now is the time to be courageous, and you will need to believe in yourself more than anybody else does. You are on this planet for one reason only: to fully step into your light and follow your heart. You get one chance at life, and it is a gift. The beauty of it is that you can choose every day, again and again, to change the course of your life's direction. If you come to finally see this, then you are truly in your power. No matter what life throws at you, you will have a strong connection to your inner wisdom and with that you can make your own decisions. But to do that, you have never needed permission from anyone.

This reminds me so vividly of a situation in my life. As I am writing this, my business is still at the beginning. It is only just becoming known. For the first time, I am making decisions that are based on my heart, and it is scary not to have anyone else's stamp of approval. My parents still don't understand what I am doing, and the chances of convincing them to understand are low as they don't speak English. Every time I tell them about a milestone achieved, their reaction is critical and not very supportive. The inner child in me sometimes takes this with compassion. I tell myself it is okay that they don't understand what I am doing and it might be even too complex to understand as they are from a different generation. I know that their reservations come from a place of love as they want the best for me and just don't see how I will make a good living from the stuff I am doing.

I don't blame them, they lived all their lives according to societal norms, but there are days where my inner child seeks and longs for their approval. Telling me that whatever I do it will work out, although they don't understand it, they have faith that it will work. But I don't get approval from them. This is exactly what I want you to be aware of.

Don't become discouraged if the people closest to you don't understand your decisions, so stop asking for their permission overall. Their life is different than yours. Their outlook on life is different than yours. And there is absolutely nothing wrong with that.

There will inevitably be days when you can cope with these moments better than others, and this chapter will prepare you for those less confident moments. When you start to feel that way, the best thing to do is find a place of stillness, where you can sit alone for at least fifteen minutes.

Get comfortable. Close your eyes. Breathe deeply, in and out a few times. Then go deep within your heart and connect with your inner child. That part within you who is longing for permission to follow through with your actions. Longing for love. While you connect with your inner child, meet yourself with your fullest compassion and a warm smile. Place your hands on your heart. Tell your inner child that it is okay to feel the way it feels. Give your inner child a hug and hold it for a while. Then look your inner child in the eyes and tell it the following:

"You don't need their permission, darling. They don't see what you see. They don't feel what you feel. But what I know for certain is, that we, you and me, want to do this because we believe in ourselves. I believe in you and I am you. We are together stronger than we think, and we will go our way. I love you deeply and together we can do this. I believe in you. I love you."

Then hug your inner child tight and notice how warm golden light from your heart is flowing into the heart of your inner child. Let this golden light fill both of you up and transmute all negative emotions into light and courage and love.

Sit in this feeling for few minutes. When you are feeling filled up with self-belief and love, you are ready to say good-bye to your inner child and come back into the now. Take one final deep breath in and out and get ready for whatever task lies ahead of you. You are filled with confidence, courage and love for who you are.

What is the essence of your most authentic self? What is it that makes you, you? What talents are you hiding? What parts of you want to come out and shine their magic? Describe that person.

· Create daily routines that support you in focusing your energy into the direction you want it to go.

· Wake up in the morning and ask yourself, what is it I want to achieve today? What do I want to spend my energy on?

· Rethink your money mind-set and come up with ways of generating income outside of the ordinary.

· Confront all the things you feel you are at war with. Where have you developed some form of resistance? Pin down your own fears, own your power.

· Visualise an inner sun in your belly to activate your solar plexus.

· Practice core exercises, high intensity training and fighting arts to balance the energy in your solar plexus out.

· Set boundaries and create distance from things that do not resonate with you. Ask yourself: do I want to be like this, or be a part of this?

· Pause throughout the day and in particular situations that might create anger or negative feelings. Ask yourself: is this part of me or my life? Does it have anything to do with me? And choose to bring your attention and energy back to the things that matter instead of letting them take control over you.

· Develop respect and understanding for others who have a different opinion and world view than you. Free yourself from the urge to seek their approval. Everybody is entitled to their opinion, and you do not need to justify your power to anyone.

· Surprise yourself by learning new things and doing things differently, break the cycle of wanting to be in control.

· Eat healing foods: eat yellow foods like lemons, bananas and complex carbs like quinoa, brown rice, oats, starchy vegetables, and legumes. Add yellow spices like curry or turmeric to your food.

Activate and balance your throat chakra

· Actively embrace your multifaceted being, explore your interests and practice self-expression.

· Work on and face your fear of rejection and fear of getting hurt.

· Embrace your talents and allow your suppressed skills to come up and unfold.

· Use your voice actively by talking, singing, and reading aloud.

· Live by your ideals and values.

· Be truthful to yourself and connect to your inner wisdom, investigate areas where you have been lying to yourself and take a new stance

· Realise that your being and what you have to give is important and relevant to this world.

· Stop comparing yourself to others and embrace being different and unique.

· Create space where you can be creative and show your uniqueness.

· Eat healing foods: blue foods like blueberry, blackberries, and blue spirulina. Also include tree fruits like apples, pears, and plums.

YOGA EXERCISES

As with the previous yoga poses you can choose to use them as a gentle flow or as Hatha yoga sequences. Do the moving poses for a total of 10 breaths in and out and hold the static poses for up to two minutes or longer.

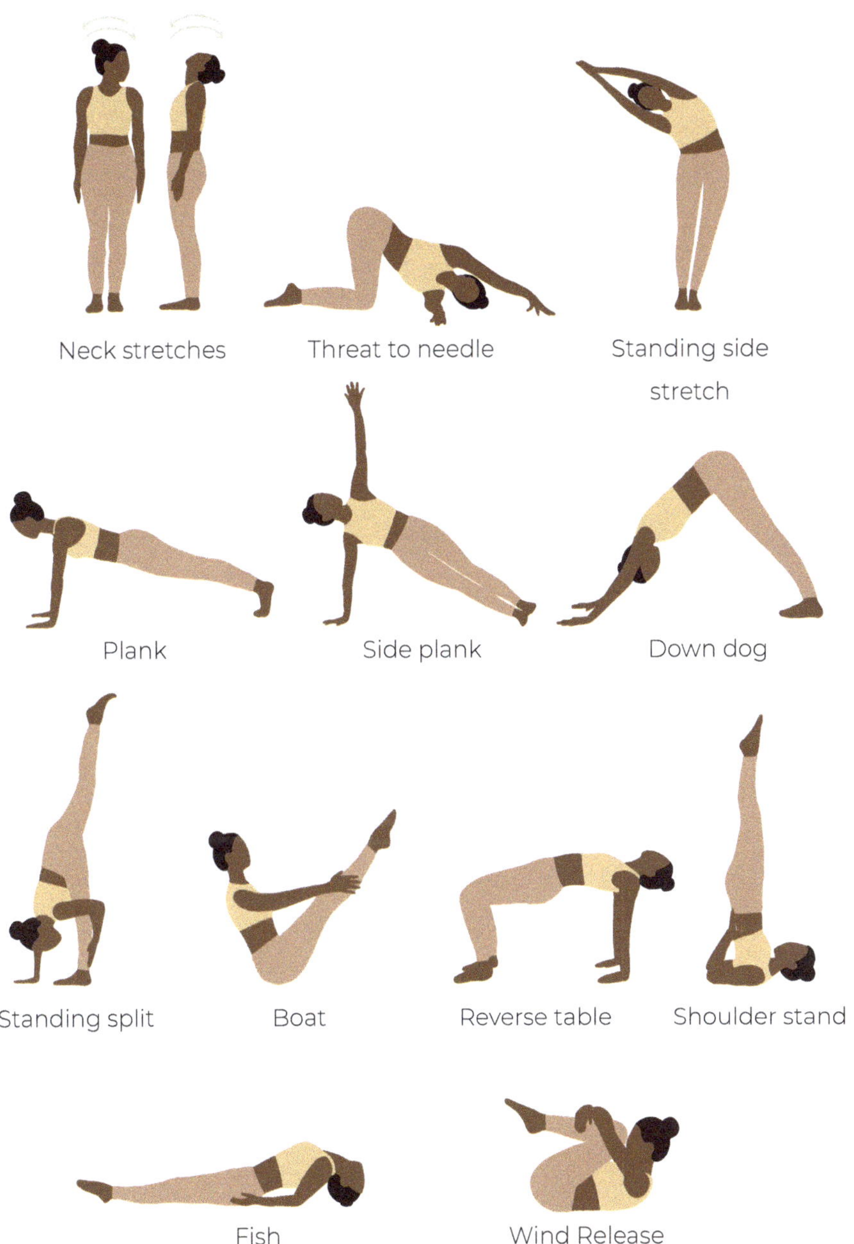

Neck stretches
Threat to needle
Standing side
stretch
Plank
Side plank
Down dog
Standing split
Boat
Reverse table
Shoulder stand
Fish
Wind Release

BREATHING EXERCISE

Sit or stand comfortably. This exercise is called four-to-seven-to-eight breathing. Breathe in through the nose and count to four. Hold your breath for seven seconds, then release through your mouth while counting to eight. It is okay if you are not immediately breathing out for eight seconds; you will improve.
Repeat this twelve times or longer if you have the time.

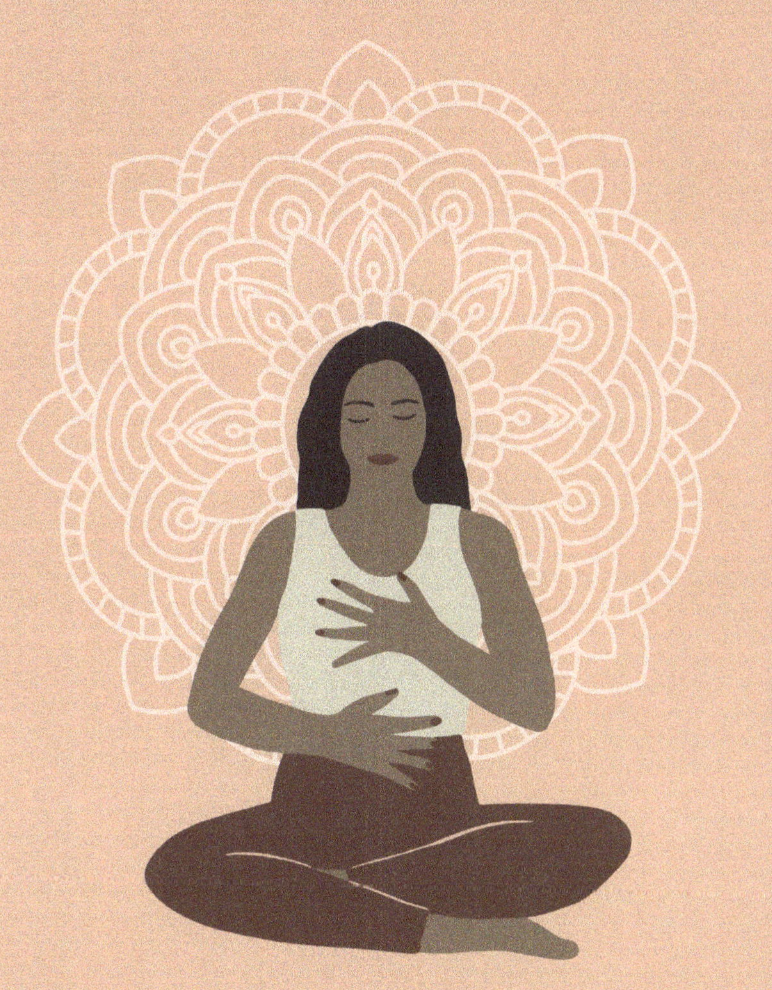

PART 5: YOUR HEART, HEALING AND YOUR SUPERPOWER

Can you imagine living a life where you follow your heart into every adventure life has to offer – and have complete trust that everything will work out? That is the power of your heart chakra.

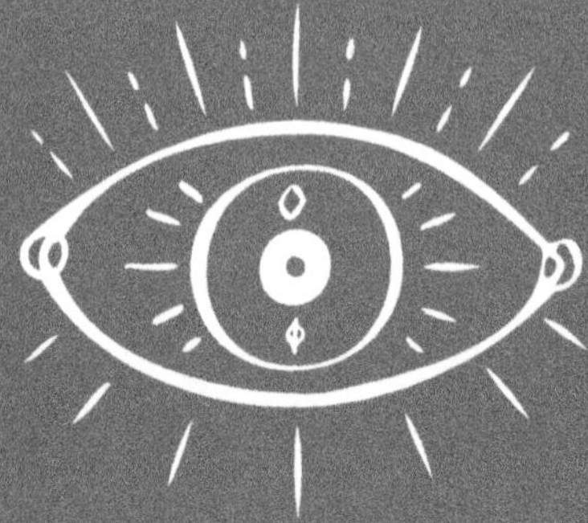

AWAKENING

When I was a child, I didn't feel I fit in. I didn't understand why kids would bully others, or me. Why teachers judged so harshly without knowing the child they were judging. I didn't understand adults behaved the way they did. Why money was such a burden, work such a stress factor, and why people were unable to speak the truth. It all was such a confusing world. People would lie to keep up a story about themselves that made them look good, but why would people do that? Why was I not allowed to wear what I wanted? Why were my parents so bothered about what others were thinking? Nothing made ever sense to me.

I also didn't understand why I could feel emotions with far more intensity than others. I remember times where strangers would open up to me, like my neighbour sitting next a 14-year-old me, telling me about her struggle with cancer. Why would people bring their worries to me, just like that? Apparently, it gave them comfort; they seemed to feel better after they left.

I didn't recognise my empath gifts fully until I started my energy healing practice. Since I was a teenager, I thought I was just hypersensitive to not just other people's emotions but also sound, light, and smells. They were so intense for me that sometimes it was too much to bear. I took lessons in psychic development and offered Reiki healing. With the first touch or connection, I could feel into the body of my clients and identify where the energetic blockages would lie. I was able to feel their pain. I realised that what I had as a child was a gift. A gift that could help people heal, but I buried it while growing up.

My life became a constant fight. A constant fight against myself. Against my body. Against money. Against my femininity. Against the government. Against everything. I treated myself poorly because I fought against the voice of my heart, because something outside, external or material was more important. I caged myself by living a life, which was leading to depression and burnout. But the whispers were there all along. The subtle feelings of knowing. The subtle whispers of guidance. My soul tried to connect and guide me, but I constantly slammed this potential deep down. Numbed it out. Ignored it. I told myself it was nonsense. I thought listening to my mind was more important than to my heart. That's the conditioning

I grew up with. The truth, however, is to trust your heart, not your mind. The HeartMath Institute published books and did research that measure our heart frequency. It found out that our heart has a 5,000 times stronger magnetic field than our brain. Meaning our heart knows things prior to our brain getting an idea of what's going on. But we grew up to live by logic, not by heart wisdom, didn't we? By 2019, the whispers and desires became louder within me, but I kept suppressing them. I didn't want to hurt others, by leaving them or disappointing them. I got used to hurting myself instead. I would see how speaking my truth would hurt others, so I thought I had better not do it.

I had a life changing week in November 2019, while my husband was travelling on business. For the first time, I was alone at home for a week. I could literally do anything I wanted. Eat when and what I wanted. Sleep in. Watch what I wanted. Do whatever made me happy without interruptions or expectations to serve. Disconnected from the world and people around me. It felt amazing. I felt like I got the chance to breathe and just be. No need to function. I even took the week off from work to enjoy myself even more. This week hit home. It was like a switch was turned inside me. Everything illuminated.

I remember feeling pure light flowing through me. Feelings of pure joy and love and understanding. I felt happier than I had ever been in my life. I was in the moment. I think of my true self shining through, aligning my energy system, but I couldn't tell you for sure exactly what it was. That week, I was guided to sign up to an energy healer course, and also signed up for yoga teacher training.

What followed was torture, because this week ended. My husband came back, and I remember I cried so badly because I didn't want to go back to this life, where my only function was to please others. But I pushed myself back into the cage, telling myself that what I must have felt was just wishful thinking. My reality was different. I was married, I was a woman with duties, I was a product manager, so I had to work, I had debts to pay.

And so, I continued for a few more months to live a life abandoning and supressing my true self. However, it all changed with my Reiki attunement. After the attunement, I felt an instant connection to higher wisdom within me, and beyond me. I had such faith in life that I knew what I had to do, and I made the tough choices. I decided to file for divorce and split from my partner, and I decided to leave my job. I had faith and so I was rewarded with an opportunity to pay off my debts and became debt-free. I was connected and somehow, I just knew what needed to be done. I received whispers of guidance, I saw visions of my future, so I took the decisions accordingly. My psychic abilities came alive, instantly connected with the source and led by my heart, and my true self fully awakened. I finally arrived home.

TOPICS COVERED BY THE HEART CHAKRA

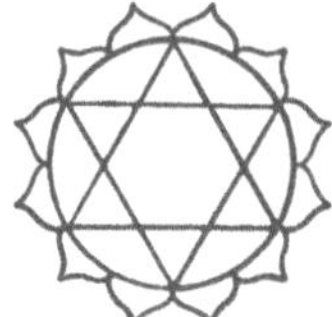

HEART CHAKRA

- Acceptance of all your parts, the lightful ones and your inner shadows.
- Sense of adventure and willingness to enjoy life to its fullest, welcome experiences – the good and the bad.
- Deep gratitude for life, for your being and everything on earth.
- Appreciation, acceptance and love for yourself.
- Welcoming change and the rhythm of life, love adventure and flexibility of life.
- See life as a game, let go of the seriousness and develop a playful attitude.

- Stop self-judgement and embrace self-compassion.
- Go new ways, do things differently than the norm, cultivate a spirit of new beginnings and be comfortable with the changes of life.
- Practice forgiveness towards others and yourself.
- Complete trust in yourself, your soul and go your heart-led way regardless of what others think or say.
- Set boundaries out of love for yourself and make yourself, your wellbeing a priority.
- Take responsibility for your own happiness and let go of co-dependency.

HEART WALLS

"And the day came when the risk it took to remain tight inside the bud was more painful than the risk it took to blossom."
Anais Nin

Have you ever come across the term heart walls? I did while undertaking training with my spiritual teacher, and then again when reading the book EMOTION CODE by Dr. Bradley Nelson. He explained the concept of heart walls from an energetic point of view.

A heart wall is basically living with a closed heart. The heart chakra is dialling down its energetic reach because you decided one day that you don't trust life, or a particular person. Hence you withdrew and created an invisible frontier around your heart chakra. One that was created as a result of hurt or trauma, through a person or situation. So, you built a heart wall towards particular people or situations.

It could be also a heart wall towards yourself, which keeps you from self-healing. And you keep this heart wall up until you finally heal the core of its origin, which you have most likely already recognised by working through this book.

When you have a closed heart or a heart wall, you are actively saying "no" to life and what life has to offer you. You are scared of being hurt, of failing, of losing something dear which makes you withdraw from the adventure and beauty life has to give. You prefer safety and aim to exist only in controlled environments. You deal with people in such a manner so you can stay in control, just to avoid pain or disappointment. We created a life with huge walls around us. We no longer allow negative experiences into our lives but at the same time this stops us allowing beautiful experiences in too. The real joys of life, they can't reach our heart centre. We dismiss feeling deeply, and only shallow feelings reach us. But our heart desires depth and it wants to experience the full spectrum of the human experience. If we close our heart, we believe that we protect ourselves from pain and hurt, but what we really do is hurt ourselves, by not allowing ourselves to feel deeply anymore, we miss out on the magical things in life.

If you allow your heart walls to fall and you stop wanting to protect yourself from life – the good and the bad – then your heart chakra becomes active. Then you will no longer care who loves you and doesn't love you. Your heart is built for rejection. It is so strong that your mind can't even comprehend its power. All your heart wants is adventure and to live the full human experience, to fall in love with life.

If you still depend on others approval in order to keep living your life, then you need to work more on your heart chakra and on vulnerability. It is not other people's role or responsibility to love you, it is your job to love yourself. With an open heart, free from guard and high walls, we allow people and experiences into our lives and allow others to heal us. Healing is the other superpower of our heart chakra.

How can you open your heart? By practising vulnerability.

Vulnerability training:

1. Love yourself and accept yourself fully.
2. Be honest to yourself.
3. Let go of the need of always having to be right.
4. Be open to learning something new, to different views and new outlooks.
5. Don't take anything personally.

When we are vulnerable, we lose the fear of the new and unknown, we lose the need to control everything and anything. We can't get hurt easily because we have learned how to deal with the unexpected, like other people's opinions. We become strong while staying soft. Just imagine that. If you are open to any experience, you lose the fear of failure because you finally understand that any experience is there for you to either learn something or enjoy something. Nothing else bad can happen. Then you realise that nothing can really hurt you. This is the beauty of letting go of the armour around your heart and opening up through your vulnerability.

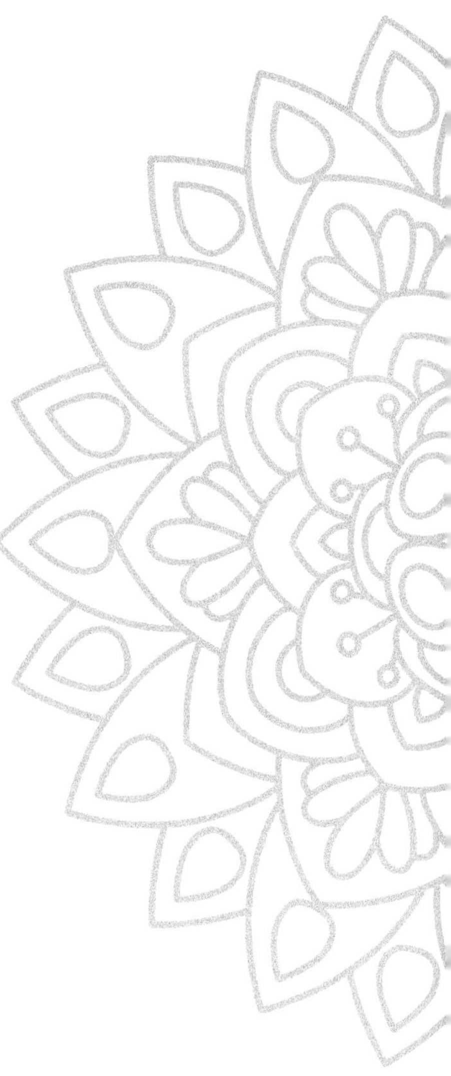

SELF-LOVE AND SELF-ACCEPTANCE

"When we were children, we learned about ourselves and about life by the reactions of the adults around us. When we grow up, we have a tendency to recreate the emotional environment of our early home life."
Louise Hay

Self-love is the key to lasting happiness, love, abundance, and everything you need. We are so disconnected with the greatness within us. So brainwashed by the outside world regarding how we need to look, how we need to live our lives, how we need to behave to be socially accepted from the start. When we were free spirits as children, we started to cage our true nature more and more with every year and every new, "You must . . . ", "You cannot . . ." etc. until we reached depression, sadness, a state of suffering and pain.

If you truly love yourself, you also respect yourself. When you respect yourself, you do not let anybody disrespect you. Nobody can hurt you because you will immediately put them in their place.

If you truly love yourself, you also take good care of yourself. When you take good care of yourself, you ensure that your energy will not become depleted by doing too much for others.

You will guard your time. You will be sure to give as much as you are comfortable with and ensure that you have enough time and energy for yourself, to regenerate, to feel good and to do the things that bring you joy.

If you truly love yourself, you speak your truth. You are honest with yourself and in doing so you don't pretend to be someone you are not. You are living in tune with your values and you are not afraid of communicating them.

If you love yourself truly, you feel capable. You have complete faith in yourself, your being and doing. You know whatever might come your way, you can handle it. You trust in your intelligence, in your strength, in you finding a solution.

Loving yourself gives you the power to create the life you truly want. You only invite people into your life who accept you as you are.

You don't allow people into your life who tell you constantly that you are wrong or that you must change. No. You don't depend on or seek the love of others because you don't need it. You are filled with love. You are all you need. Therefore, self-love is a major step to becoming your true self. Loving and accepting yourself the way you look, the way you think, and the way you are.

Most importantly, you deserve love and a fulfilling and magical love relationship. Don't believe anything less. In order to have a fulfilling love relationship, you have to love yourself fully and accept your greatness. It is said that once you love yourself, only then will you attract the right person to your life.

However, I also believe that if you love yourself only 60% instead of fully 100%, you can still attract the right person. A partnership can help us love ourselves and heal and accept ourselves with lightning speed, but only in a healthy way. Because if your partner can love you, the true you, all the parts you don't love about yourself, all the parts you deem weird or too much of something, then you can learn to love yourself and all those parts, too.

However, if you are in a partnership where you are constantly being made to feel wrong and that the way you look, or the way you are, is not good enough, then trust that you are clearly in the wrong relationship. A mismatch. I believe in matches. There is someone for you out there who fits to you like no other. Once I found my match, it was like having found a magnifier of self-love. I am being cherished for my weird parts of speaking, of connecting to spirits, feeling tree energy, love of self-defence arts, seeing and feeling light beings and the power of energy healing. He loves that about me. And I can finally accept the childish parts of me. Being weak after years of only being strong. Accepting my body whole-heartedly although I do not look like a fitness model.

This is the power of healing past trauma with a true love re-lationship. You don't have to wait until you fully love yourself. It is a journey. But a real match can support you as much as you might support the other half. So don't tell yourself you are not ready for a new relationship because you don't love yourself fully. It is okay. A word of warning though. I have de-scribed a healthy relationship so far, but be aware that if you become addicted to constant confirmation and validation by your partner, this is very unhealthy. It is no longer healing, but self-destructive.

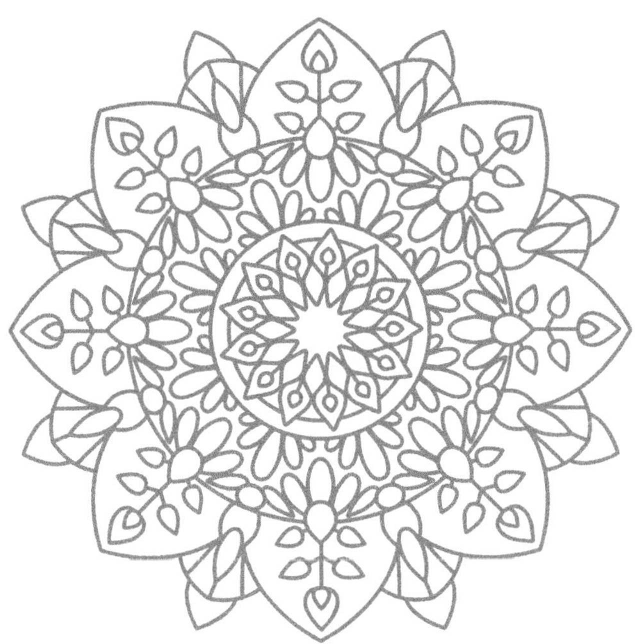

WELCOME TO YOUR DARK SIDE – YOUR INNER SHADOWS

What are our inner shadows?

They are parts of us that we repress, that we don't accept and we do not allow ourselves to be. Like being vulnerable, weak, childish, etc. They are based on experiences in our life, when one day we came to the conclusion that we don't allow ourselves to be a particular way.

Maybe because our parents told us not to be dreamers or childish. To all the men out there, how often did you hear the phrase "boys don't cry"? At work we were told that being lazy will get you fired. Maybe our first love told us that we suck in bed and so we don't allow and accept our sexual needs but rather suppress them. Those are our inner shadows. They are hidden within us but still working subconsciously against us. This is why it is so important for us to accept them. To accept all parts of ourselves and who we are. Because, trust me, we cannot love ourselves fully, cannot build our best life and bring our truest self to the surface if we don't allow ourselves to be who we want to be. There will be moments when you will be lazy and that's okay; you need to rest sometimes as well. There will be moments when you will be emotional, childish, creative, weak, strong, etc. This is part of life. Each emotion and each behaviour is based on polarity – and you have all of them within you. The ones, however, that shine through depend on your inner radio station.

All of those emotions are parts of you. You, however, decide the extent in which you tune into them. If you, let's say, are confident and always act mature and work very hard without giving yourself a break, you might have some very great attributes. But do you see the costs? You don't rest. You don't play. You don't have fun. Where is the joy in that? Suppose you have a low moment like, let's say, being fearful. Trust that you can change the channel on your inner radio station by changing your thoughts and feelings and tune into love. Because love is part of you as much as being fearful. All parts of you are beneficial at different moments. They are all part of you. So do not reject them. Accept them.

- What parts of yourself don't you like and accept? What parts do you believe you are not allowed to be? Which do you feel ashamed of?
- Why do you not accept this part of you? What would happen if you accepted this part?
- How can those parts, your inner shadows benefit your life? What gift could they bring?

Allow yourself to live all the parts within you. They are a part of you. Forgive yourself for not accepting them. You are whole already. Don't make yourself smaller than you are. Love all of yourself.

How can you identify your shadows throughout the day? Afterall, there are a lot of parts of you that will come out over the years. Well, the fastest way to encounter a shadow is when someone else is displaying a behaviour that triggers you. For example, a former boss of mine annoyed me. She didn't understand the business process, the product, or anything at all. However, instead of doing the sensible thing and asking questions and learning, she covered her lack of knowledge with bitchiness. This, of course, made the team's work life harder. Now, what exactly triggered me? Someone doesn't know something and covers it with ego behaviour is a sign of insecurity. So, this was one part of me I didn't allow to come up or I didn't want to display. I hated the feeling of insecurity so much that it triggered me seeing it in others. Back then, I also lived under the mask of being a strong woman, and I considered insecurity a weakness – which was then an inner shadow of mine.

Once you have identified your inner shadow you can use the questions above to integrate it. A shortcut would be these two steps:

- **Step 1:** accept there is a gift behind your shadow.
- **Step 2:** accept that part of you regardless of if you find a gift behind it or not. Close your eyes, place your hands on your heart chakra. Take three deep belly breaths in and out. Say to yourself: "(name the shadow part) although I can't find any gift behind your being, I love and accept you. I let you now into

my heart. You are a part of me, and I love you regardless." Then envision how your heart chakra is shining bright, hugging your inner shadow and integrating it into your heart. Stay there for as long as you need to feel it being integrated in your system.

Why is it so important to accept all parts of us? Because 50% of your personal power and manifestation source comes from your dark side – your shadows. Sometimes you might have manifested something, but you couldn't keep it. Or you tried to manifest it, but it didn't happen. This could be because your shadow manifested with you. And there is or was one part within you that was stronger and manifested the opposite. This is why it is so important on so many levels to make peace with your shadows and integrate them into your system. Unconditional acceptance, especially of parts like being fearful, not good enough, or undeserving can impact our manifestation power and overall success and well-being on so many levels.

The power of your heart chakra is love. This means it encompasses everything including fear, hate and all the things you might regard as negative. Love can transmute them all. Making the way free for love means making the way free for life to reach you.

FORGIVENESS

"The weak can never forgive. Forgiveness is an attribute of the strong."
Mahatma Gandhi

No effort is as difficult as forgiveness, whether it be forgiving yourself or forgiving others; however, nothing opens the heart faster than forgiveness. Nothing will allow you to love yourself more than forgiveness. Nothing but forgiveness allows you to say goodbye to your emotional baggage and feel light again. Nothing besides forgiveness will set you free. Forgiveness is the greatest gift you can give yourself.

Forgiveness means healing. Remorse, holding on to the past, is one of the major reasons for our suffering today. People who tend to think about the past, who relive it over and over again, keep suffering. We are the only beings on Earth who freely choose to pay for our mistakes a million times by thinking and reliving our past over and over again. You can't change your past, you can only accept it and let go, so you can take your power back, allowing you to live in the now. Life is created in the moment, in the now, not by reliving the past, or thinking about the future.

Begin the forgiveness process with yourself.

- What are you not forgiving yourself for? What past experiences are weighing on you?
- What could you learn from that experience? What did you learn about yourself?
- Who can you be today because of that experience?
- Who would you be today without that experience?

Take some time to reflect on those questions and if you feel like it, write a forgiveness letter.

Forgiving others is equally important. This does not mean that you agree with what they did. No, absolutely not. But what you are doing by forgiving them is cutting lose the baggage you're carrying. Set yourself free to live a truly love-filled and joyful life. There are so many cases of illnesses that could be healed through forgiveness and balancing your energy system. Illnesses can manifest as blocked energy from holding on to resentment. Cancer of the ovaries for example when we reject our femininity or don't forgive wrongdoing related to sexuality in women. Cancer or lung disease if we hold on to pain from the past with emotions of anger or grief. And so many more illnesses where forgiveness can release the energy blockage and allow space for healing. I advise you to write a letter to each person. You don't have to send the letters. It is the process of letting it all out, saying all the things you could never say or were too afraid to say. Blame them, get angry, let all your pain and frustration out when writing it all out. Write the letter to release your resentment, and then destroy the letter. Then it is done. Gone. Out of your life. Recognise the price of your blame and become aware of its impact on how you are living. Answer the following questions:

- Against whom do you hold resentment?
- What should never have happened in your life?
- If I keep holding on to those accusations, then what will happen?
- What would happen if you let go of them? Who would you be? How would your life be without them? What would be different?

After writing your forgiveness letter, it is important to realise the learning that you can take from those painful experiences. I know it sounds wrong, but each painful experience was a huge learning curve for you. Trust me.

Tony Robbins, one of the greatest life coaches of our time if you ask me, said once to blame intelligently. If you blame a person for all the bad they did to you, blame them also for all the good that came out of that. I know it sounds like a very foreign concept at first. Somebody hurt you how shall that be something positive. But let's be honest if your parents didn't show you love, you learned to survive without it, you became stronger. If you were cheated by your partner, you could come to learn and understand their betrayal. You might have since learned how to identify signs when people are not true with you. But you could only come to this because you had to go through the process of being cheated on and lied to. Every person who harms us makes us stronger in some way. Just think about how much power this knowledge gives you.

Therefore, I want you to take the time to write down, for each of those people you need to forgive, the lessons you could gain from the hurt they caused you. What were you able to overcome? How did you overcome it? Did you become stronger? Did you realise the strength and intelligence within you? Did it make you find your voice and speak up for yourself? Did it empower you to finally stand up for yourself?

YOUR PAST IS YOUR STRENGTH

Major life experiences forced you to grow and become stronger. We need to fall in order to rise. Be weak in order to become strong. Experience pain in order to experience love. Know sadness in order to experience happiness. Be betrayed in order to appreciate honesty. Get hurt in order to feel com-passion. Be broke in order to value wealth. Feel fear in order to become confident. Get sick in order to heal and appreciate health. Fail in order to learn. Feel numb in order to value coming fully into our life. Where there is darkness there is light. Hatred there is love. Fear there is joy. Wherever you are, full potential is at your fingertips. Within you.

YOU ARE A CREATOR

Do you see the power you hold? Did you come to understand how powerful your truly are? That you are a creator? You don't owe this world anything. You only owe it to yourself to live a life worth living – to your standards and personal wellbeing. Your health and happiness come first. There are so many books, blogs, podcasts on the topic of the law of attraction. They simply say: what you give out comes back to you. So, if you send out negativity, you get it back in some way. If you send out positivity you will receive positivity.

You have experienced it already. Remember the days when you got up and everything that could go wrong, went wrong? And on the other hand, there are days where you get up in the morning and everything just works out brilliantly, good news, extra money, kind words etc. That's the law of attraction at work. For it to work in your favour, you don't have to be in a positive mind state all day, every day. All you need is to ensure for at least 51% of the day you are in a more positive state than negative.

Another famous example of the law of attraction was Jim Carrey.

In 1985, Jim Carrey wrote himself a $10 million cheque for "acting services rendered," and dated it ten years in the future. He carried it with him at all times in his wallet. In November 1995, a miraculous thing happened. Call it a coincidence, but Carrey found out he was casted for the movie Dumb and Dumber where he was paid $10 million.

There are many more examples out there and if I think about my own life, I manifested the money to pay off my debts, I manifested my dream partner and dream life. I am saying to you that you are a creator, and you can literally manifest and create your dream life no matter what. But for this to happen, you need to open up to life and let go of trying to control everything and following the requests and expectations of others. Instead, open up to life and let your heart and inner wisdom guide you. The magic that comes into your life will blow you away.

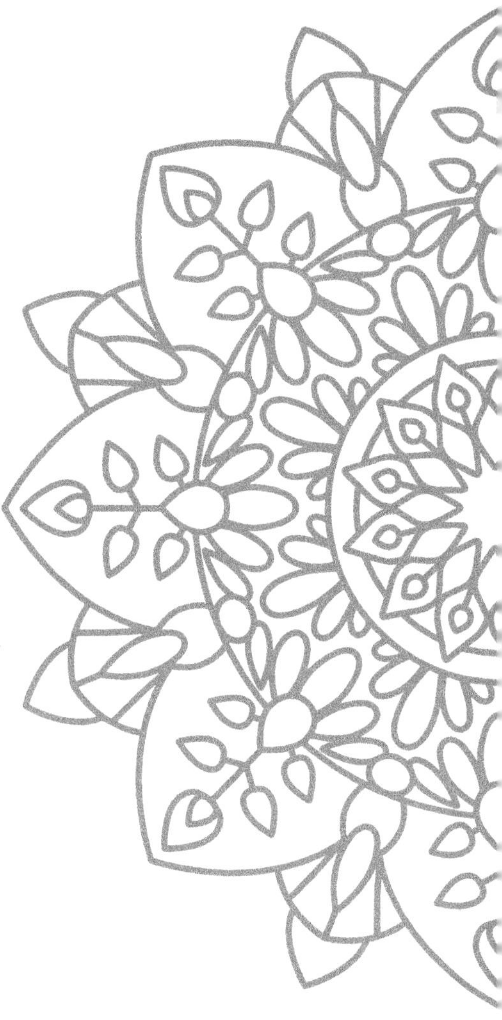

SHINE - YOUR LIFE IS YOUR MESSAGE

"When you step into your power and your true authentic self. You shine. You shine so brightly that the world tries to keep up."
Shannon Kaiser

Gandhi once said, "my life is my message". Same goes with you. What do you want to stand for? What expression shall your life be? What is it that you want to be remembered for? For being funny? For living your life on your own terms? For being a successful artist? No matter what your heart calls you to do or be, it is valid. You have a message to share with the world and living a life that is not sharing your message is selfish because others might depend on your message and light. You are on this earth for a reason. And this reason is not to suffer, but instead awaken to your full potential and live according to your heart.

You have undertaken quite a journey already with this book. You are all set and ready to create your dream life. Something, I was missing while on my own personal journey of healing and transformation. No self-help book offered me guidance, nor were the people around me. The tough moments along the journey, that make you doubt everything you are and do will arise. But they will lessen over time as you live every day more and more as the true version of yourself. However, in the beginning they may occur more often than you expect and guess what? That is totally normal.

There will be moments of doubt, of pain, of the past, of limiting beliefs that might reoccur. When I decided to divorce from my partner I struggled with past memories flooding my system unexpectedly. There were times during my professional career steps when I was filled with doubt and fear, wondering if I was really doing the right thing. Who am I to do all that I desire? Who am I to follow my heart for the first time since I was a child? Such moments can arise, especially when our surroundings are telling us that we are crazy to do something different. After all, it takes courage and utter faith in ourselves and life. I learned something important. When people think you are completely crazy and whatever you do is wrong, then trust that you definitely do the right thing. Greatness never comes from doing the same as everyone else does.

LIONHEART: YOUR HEART AND COURAGE

"Our deepest fear is not that we are inadequate. Our deepest fear is that we are powerful beyond measure. It is our Light, not our Darkness, that most frightens us."
Marianne Williamson

Everything you go for in your life, especially when it is about following your dreams, requires heart and courage. So, remember every time you are on your way to do something new, or your heart is called to do something, you are activating the bravest version of you. Not only that, but you are also sending your courage to others to do the same. You become the role model that they seek. Too many people don't act out of fear and limiting self-belief. People might try and bring you down because they don't want to see you succeed, simply because they would love to do the same, but they are too scared to take the first step. But you are doing it and that takes heart and courage.

Every time you do something new, trust that it is worth it and believe in yourself. You wouldn't have thought about it if you weren't ready for it. That's how simple it is. When you look around and see people already doing what you desire to do, then trust you can do it. You can only see it that skill or attribute because it is already within you. As the full potential of a rose is within a seed, so is your full potential available within yourself to become the person you desire to be.

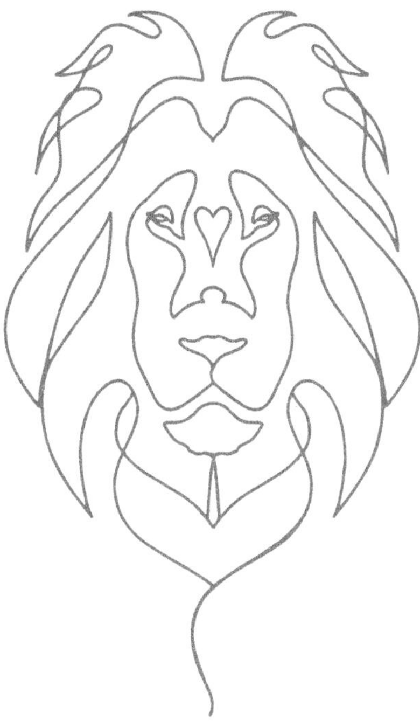

HEALING IS A LIFELONG JOURNEY

If you believe that healing and personal transformation is something like a goal, that once you achieve it you are done or complete, I have to tell you that will never happen as long as you live. Trust that once you are no longer growing and learning or developing as a person that this comes close to you stopping your life, putting it on hold.

Life is an adventure and once you say yes to it, it is like a rollercoaster of great and amazing experiences. There will be ups and downs and we need those in order to heal and transform and change as a person.

Change is beautiful. It keeps us alive, transforming, learning, becoming better and wiser.

Does that mean we will not do something semi-great? Of course we will. We might also have a bad day and say something stupid to our partner or parent. Apologise and move on. We will experience tough circumstances and tough choices but this is part of life too. While you are on your journey you might every once and a while remember moments from the past that were not pretty, but this just means there is still something left you can let go of. Something left to heal and to learn.

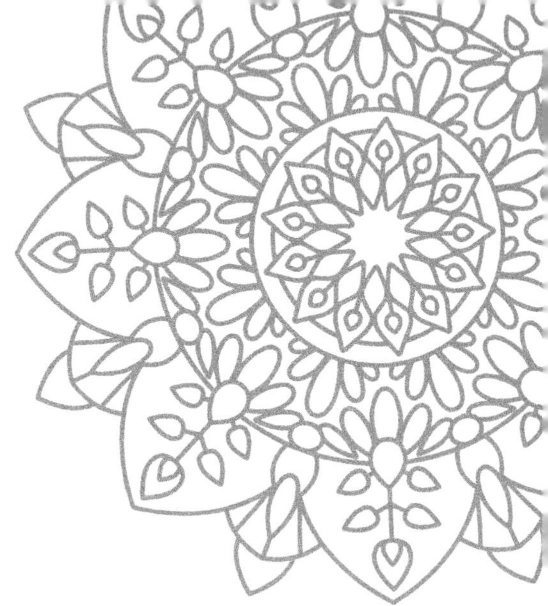

Healing is a journey. If your dad caused you a major trauma in your childhood, you might have to repeat some forgiveness or re-read your letter about what you are grateful for again in order to let go of that last bit of remorse. Sometimes you don't know even why but you feel like crying, and it feels like a burden from the past. The best thing you can do, instead of overthinking and over questioning whatever is coming up, is to actually let it go. Cry if needed. Write it out. Sing, scream, run. Whatever you are called to do, just do it and let it go. We do not need to know what and why exactly, although our brain would like to figure it out. But sometimes all we need to do is allow the emotion or memory to surface, so we can say a last goodbye and let it flow and let it go.

· Inner parts or shadow work and accepting yourself with everything you are.

· Forgiveness work especially towards yourself.

· Letting go instead of holding on to things, people or situations.

· Heart wall release and allowing yourself to flow with life, vulnerability.

· Openness to adventure and doing new things, while having faith that everything works out the way it should, be more flexible and spontaneous.

· Interrupt self-judging thoughts and self-harming behaviour, instead show up for yourself with love and compassion.

· Chest opening asanas from yoga, expanding your heart centre.

· Pranayama exercises, breathing deeply and feeling into your heart centre.

· Question paradigms and rules of what is good and what is bad, what is beautiful what is ugly, and let go of things that are no longer in line with your own beliefs and views.

• Observe and interrupt your own self-judging cycle – show yourself compassion and understanding.

• Don't make your happiness dependent of others, love without expectations.

• Strength and cardio training that improves your heart rate variability.

• Practice daily gratitude.

• Be open to new things and try new things out

• Accept what can't be changed. Accept limitations but don't let them rule your life. Accept but still live a life to your full potential, do the things that you are called to do.

• Eat healing food, especially green ones. Ideally make it 30-40% of your diet. Include green beans, broccoli, kale, spinach, avocado, kiwi, cucumber, courgette, and others daily.

YOGA EXERCISES

As with the previous yoga poses you can choose to use them as a gentle flow or as Hatha yoga sequences. Do the moving poses for a total of 10 breaths in and out and hold the static poses for up to two minutes or longer.

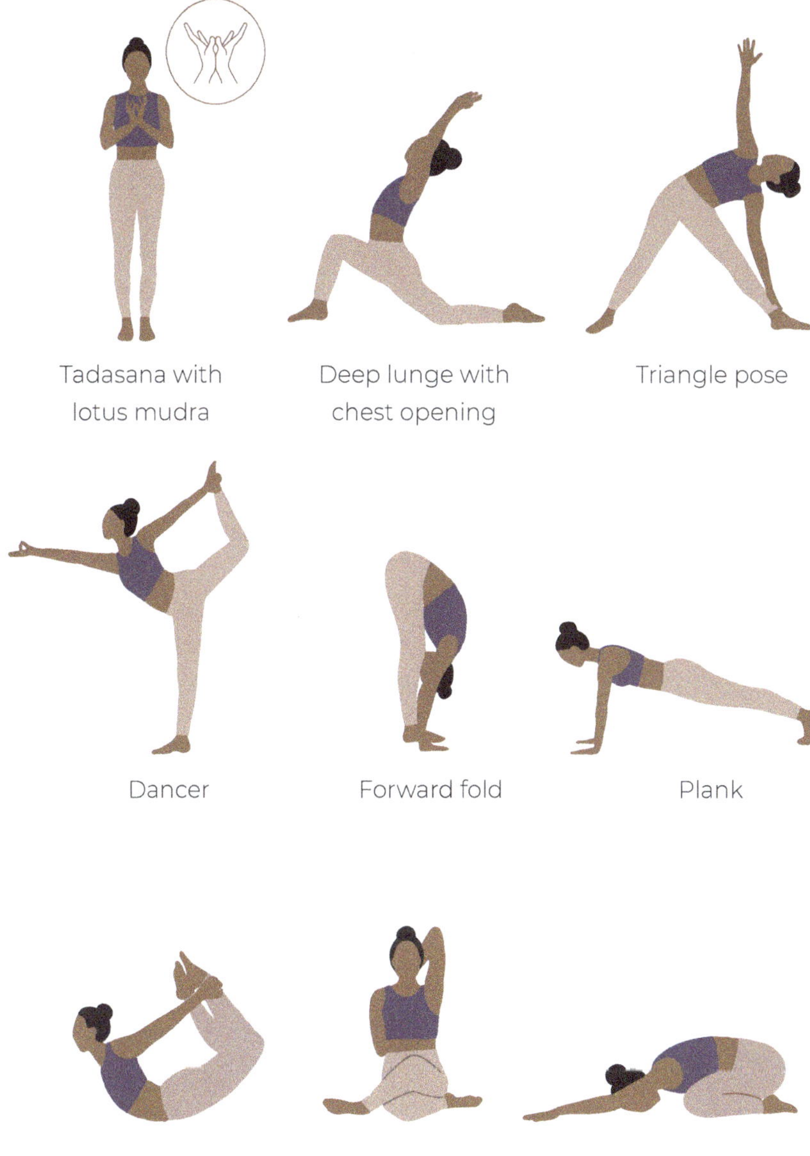

Tadasana with lotus mudra

Deep lunge with chest opening

Triangle pose

Dancer

Forward fold

Plank

Bow

Cow face

Child pose

MEDITATION

This is a mediation for heart light, and it should take 15 minutes.

Find a comfortable position where you can sit, either on a chair, a cushion, a pillow or on your bed. You can lean your back on the wall for support if you like.

Then sit upright, shoulders away from your ears but comfortable in your position. Bring your attention to your body and where it is touching the chair, the floor, or your cushion. Focus on your sensations and just feel into your body. Start breathing deeply. Bring your attention to your chest and your belly. Feel how they rise when you breathe in and how they flatten out when you breathe out. Try to be with each breath for its full duration. You might start to notice your mind wandering off. When you notice this, just come back and focus on your breathing. It is okay for your mind to start wandering off. Every time this happens just bring it back by focusing on your breathing.

Keep breathing deeply in and out, with your focus and attention on how your chest and belly is rising and falling. Then bring your attention to your heart centre, your heart chakra. Imagine there is a golden light ball there. With every inhale this light ball become bigger and bigger. Continue breathing until the light ball has grown so big that it literally surrounds you. Visualise how the light from your heart centre is flowing through your veins, your body, into your cells, transmuting everything that is not 100% positive into light. Blockages dissolved. Negativity dissolved. Only pure white golden light flowing through you as you. Continue to breathe and bathe in this light that comes from your heart chakra healing and balancing your whole being. Stay as long as it feels good for you in this meditation. When you end this practice, become aware of the now and slowly open your eyes.

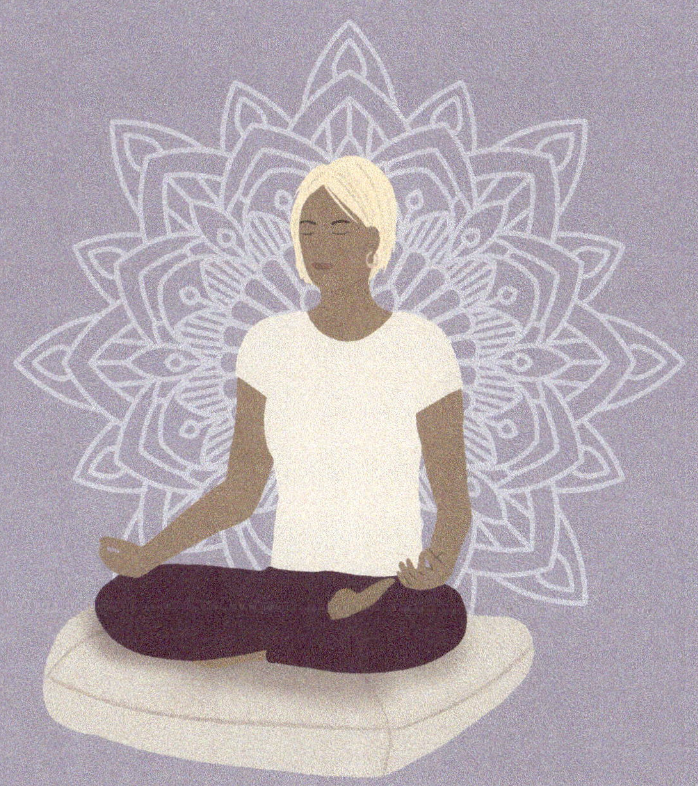

PART 6:
THE ARRIVAL OF YOU

I no longer allow anybody or anything to dim my light. I am light. My purpose is to shine. That is my mission.

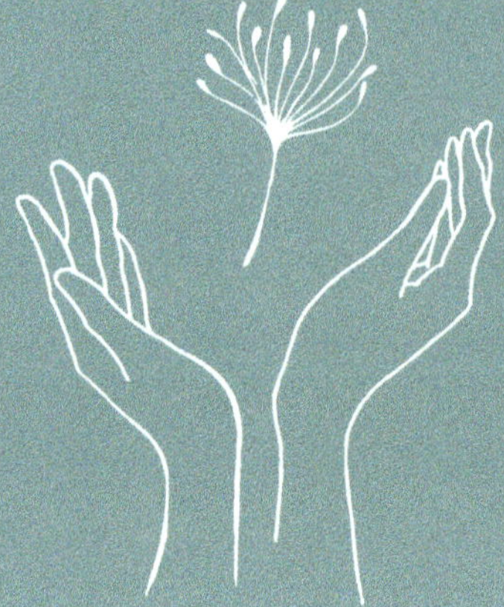

THE GIFT WITHIN YOU

This is the story of the gift hidden within you, a short Hindu tale.

In one of our yoga philosophies classes, my yoga teacher told an amazing tale:

There was a time on Earth where all human beings were in fact gods. All had a special gift. However, people started to abuse their godly power and thus the God of Gods Brahman decided to take this power away from humankind. On that particular day, he held a council meeting with his other Gods to discuss the matter and decide where to hide their powers. One of the other gods suggested to hide their gifts deep in the sea so they would never be found. However, Brahman denied.

"There will come a day that mankind will find a way to conquer the sea and will be able to find it," he said.

Another God suggested to hide their gifts at the deepest point of Earth. But also, Brahman denied it.

"There will come a day where mankind will find a way to break open the deepest point of the Earth, it is not safe there," he said.

Another God suggested the far universe as a place to hide their gifts. Brahman was still not convinced.

"There will be a time where mankind will find ways to enter the universe and will be able to find it. This is still not a safe place," he said.

The Gods were confused. "So, there is no land, no sea, no space where we can hide their powers. What shall we do then?"

Brahman had a brilliant idea: "I know where to hide it. We will hide it deep within their heart centre. Mankind will never be able to find it there."

The other gods agreed. And so, it was done.

You are a god. Once you connect back to your true self, to your heart, you find your superpower, and nothing can stop you anymore.

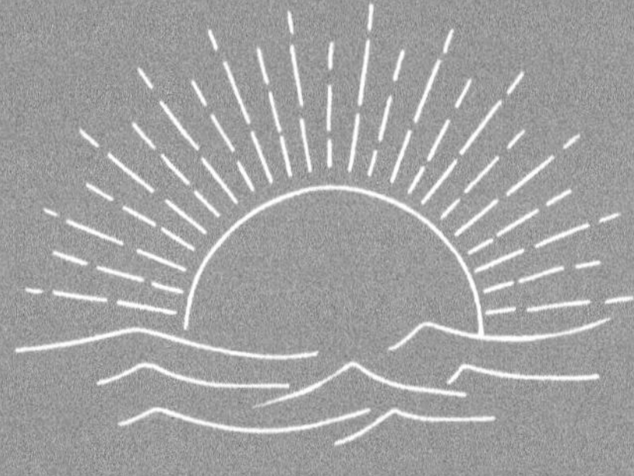

An old man was walking after a storm had passed along the beach. Fishes were lying on the beach unable to get into water. The old man saw a little boy throwing one fish after the other back into the sea. The old man asked the little boy:

"Son, what are you doing?"

The little boy looked at him for a moment and then continued throwing one fish after the other into the sea.

"I help the fishes to get back into the water, Sir," the boy replied.

The old man shook his head and said, "Don't waste your time, you cannot save them all."

The little boy carried on saving one fish after another and replied, "I might not be able to save them all, but for this one," and he threw one fish into the sea, "it made a difference."

Like the little boy from this story, you and me, and all who start following their heart make a difference. Even if it is small, together we make a huge difference to our lives and also to the lives of others. We contribute to the better and the more we are true to ourselves, the healthier and happier we become, and the more we light up this world we live in.

If Burnout taught me one major lesson, it is that the best you can do for your physical, mental, emotional, and spiritual health is to be your true self. Being yourself is the greatest gift you can give yourself and this world. Be the light tower.

With this, I wish you all the best for the future. May you shine your light and come out of that place your soul is hiding and light up this world with your uniqueness.

Always remember, no one is like you, and that is your superpower.

With love,
Claudia

GRATITUDE

Thank you to the editors at House of Editors in London especially Marcus for liaising and the support of finding the right editor for this project. Thank you, Becky Milroy, for your dedication, critical feedback and support in editing this book. Thank you for your expertise and time you put into it.

Special thanks to Irene, a magical design artist who created the design for this book inside out. You created such beauty and I thank you so much for empowering the words I wrote with your visual design and illustrations.

Thank you to my spiritual teachers, healers and people who supported me with their wisdom in my personal growth. My yoga teachers must foremost Sarah Lo, for her mind-blowing and transformative teachings. Your teacher trainings just levelled up my mindfulness skills to new highs, not to mention my personal development. Thank you to all my Reiki teachers. Your light and wisdom sparked my light.

Special thanks to my heart-soul people. Most and foremost thank you Lukas, for your unconditional love and support in everything I do, no matter how crazy my ideas sometimes get. Thank you for your relentless support throughout my own personal crisis and healing journey. I wouldn't be where I am today without you. I love you.

Danke, dass es dich gibt, Denisa, ohne dich wäre mein Weg
nicht ganz so leicht verlaufen. Deine Unterstützung, deine Kraft,
dein Herz und Verständnis gaben mir dir Kraft mir selbst zu
helfen. Danke dir! Ich hab dich lieb.

Thank you to my special friend, Magdalena. Although you are
rooted on the other side of the globe, I am so grateful for knowing you. Without your support and wisdom during my darkest
hour I wouldn't have been able to make it through the way I did.
I am utmost grateful for having you in my life.

Danke dir Lena! Wir haben uns wieder gefunden, zu einer Zeit,
wo wahre Freundschaft zur Mangelware für mich wurde. Doch
du brachtest mir Zuversicht, Hoffnung und Mut meinen Weg zu
gehen. Und das schönste ist, du bist noch immer da! Danke dir
für dein sein! Du bist wunderbar!

Thank you, Ayllin, you reminded me for who I am actually writing
this book. I met you and I found the younger version of me in you.
Strong, with a big heart and so much genuine love. I thank you
for being and your support as friend. Although it might not been
my first intention, as I didn't know you yet. But this book is for you.
Reading through it in the final end stages, I can whole heartedly
say, this is for you my dear. May it bring you courage for your light.

Danke Mama und Papa, für eure Liebe und auch wenn ich man-
chmal ein Mysterium für euch bin, ihr mich dennoch machen
lässt, wonach mein Herzilein mich ruft. Ich hab euch ganz doll lieb!

ABOUT THE AUTHOR

Claudia is a certified Yoga teacher, Reiki Master, Energy Healer, and Mindfulness Coach. Currently she is based in Prague, where she offers Reiki Sessions and Teacher trainings. Her utmost goal is to support people to come back home to their true self and start living a life in congruence to their heart's desire. Her overall 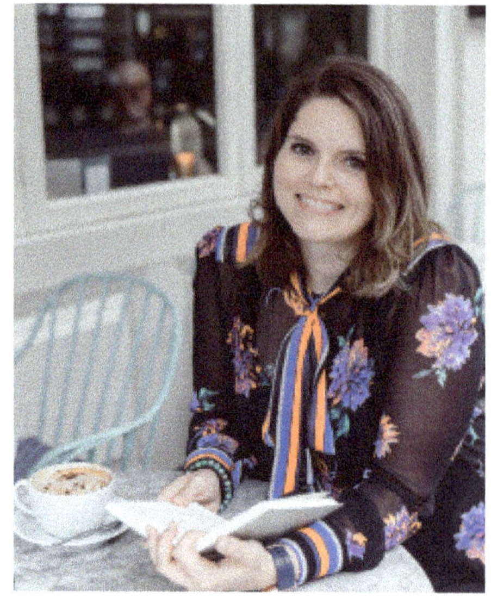 mission is to fight stress worldwide and offer her clients and students tools to come into their essence, break free from societal conditioning and live a healthy and soul-led life - A TRUE SELF ACTIVIST.

After suffering herself in 2020 from severe burnout her mission is to provide help to people who need immediate anti-stress therapy and support. She focuses heavily on a holistic health approach with special attention to the energy body and energy healing modalities such as Reiki, Trance Healing, Yoga, and Spiritual Coaching.

Since she was a child, she could sense and feel other people's feelings and emotions. Throughout her life she helped transform people's life by empowering and supporting them in personal development and following their heart. Claudia is passionate to use the experience of her own life and her natural abilities to help others heal mentally, emotionally, and spiritually.

FURTHER READING AND RESOURCES

- *The Power* by Rhonda Byrne
- *You Are a Badass* by Jen Sincero
- *A New World* by Eckhart Tolle
- *The Four Agreements* by Don Miguel Ruiz
- *Breaking the Habit of Being Yourself* by Dr. Joe Dispenza
- *Warrior Goddess Training: Become the Woman You Are Meant to Be* by Heatherash Amara
- *You Can Heal your Life* by Louise Hay
- *Light is the New Black* by Rebecca Campbell
- *Loving What Is: Four Questions that Can Change Your Life* by Byron Katie
- *Awaken the Giant Within* by Tony Robbins

GET IN TOUCH

www.claudiaandreareiter.com
@trueselfcalling
Fb: Claudia Andrea Reiter
Email: hello@claudiaandreareiter.com

Heal with me:
Reiki healing (distant or in person)
Chakra Assessment (distant or in person)
Reiki & Yoga Retreat
Info on: www.claudiaandreareiter.com/heal-with-me

Train with me:
Become a Psychic Reiki Healer

www.ingramcontent.com/pod-product-compliance
Lightning Source LLC
LaVergne TN
LVHW051117180726
843512LV00012B/863